Natural Pet Healing

NATURAL PET HEALING

Our Psychic, Spiritual Connection

Von Braschler

2003
Galde Press, Inc.
Lakeville, Minnesota, U.S.A.

Printed in the United States of America

First Edition
First Printing, 2003

Cover photograph Alyssa Friesen and cairn terrier puppy Olga.
Interior photographs courtesy of Cynthia McNeill.
Interior drawings and illustrations by Sarah Andersen.

Library of Congress Cataloging-in-Publication Data

Braschler, Von, 1947-
Natural pet healing : our psychic, spiritual connection / Von Braschler.
p. cm.
Includes bibliographical references.
ISBN 1-9319-07-2 (trade pbk)
1. Pets--Diseases--Alternative treatment. 2. Holistic veterinary medicine. 3. Spiritual healing. I. Title.
SF981 .B73 2003
636.089'55--dc22
2003020393

Galde Press, Inc.
PO Box 460
Lakeville, Minnesota 55044–0460

To Wizard and Deb,

united in spirit.

Contents

Introduction

Healing Pets, Plants, and Yourself

The history of empathic healing is rich with stories of symbiotic relationships between people and other animals. There is even a healthy symbiotic relationship between our pets and plants and between people and their houseplants. Indeed, we can heal each other with our healing touch, our energized thought forms, and other methods of transferring energy from one life form to another.

Empathic healing goes by many names. It has been called everything from bodywork to healing hands, massage, energy healing, psychic healing, magnetic healing, touch therapy, therapeutic touch, reiki, and chakra therapy. The labels we give it matter very little. What matters is the way natural healing allows us to connect effectively to make a difference.

This is possible because all of life is interconnected and interdependent. With compassion and a little training, it is relatively easy for any of us to reach out and touch other lives, to energize them and restore their health and well-being.

In this book, I will show you how to use your hands, your head, and your heart to heal those near and dear to you. This could include a loved animal who shares your life. It could include a houseplant or tree in your yard. It could even include yourself.

This is not a magical illusion or sleight of hand. We will employ time-honored principles to produce and transfer the sort of energy that you will require for natural healing. In the end, you will see that this principle is just as natural as a mother's healing kiss on a skinned elbow—and just as effective. It is as natural as the gentle rain or sun that restores life all around us in nature.

Nothing in this book is meant to serve as a substitute for professional medical attention for those in need of immediate care. Nor do I advocate using any of these natural healing techniques in place of proper veterinary care or the help of botanical experts. A sick dog or a sick plant deserves the very best care we can provide, and that means professional care.

The self-healing techniques in this book can be used as a supplement to professional care. None of these techniques contradict or counteract the care provided by medical professionals. Rather, our natural healing techniques are meant to complement the treatment of medical professionals by energizing the patient to begin the healing process.

All healing comes from within. All living things are self-regenerative. Consequently, the patient heals himself or herself. All that any of us can do is to help that natural process. Treatment is not healing. Treatment simply assists the body of the injured party to begin the self-healing process.

This is folk healing as old as human compassion. It was practiced before there was an organized medical profession with doctors and hospitals. It has proven its worth by standing the test of time. It is natural. It recognizes the value and well-being of all life.

All life is sacred and precious. Every individual life matters in the grand scheme of things and contributes significantly to the harmony of all. This includes every animal and every plant. Remove any songbird, and the great symphony of the universe is diminished. Eliminate even the smallest wildflower, and the beautiful pattern of life is broken. Indeed, all of life is connected and mutually dependent. We are all interrelated. Together, we form the whole.

And so our health is interrelated in the perfect balance of nature. A person breathes oxygen that is discharged from a tree and then expels carbon dioxide to nourish the tree. This typifies the interdependent cycle of life. A human being pets a dog or cat, giving that pet a healing touch that fosters well-being. In turn, that act of kindness creates a calming effect upon the person, reducing stress, blood pressure, and risk of heart problems and other ailments.

Pets and plants have been incorporated into many therapy programs for people, as the natural health benefits of interspecies communication and cooperation have become more widely acknowledged. Now empathic healing shows how people can affect the well-being of our pets and plants with natural healing that transfers personal energy from body to body.

This is mutually beneficial. As we heal those around us, we become well ourselves. The circle of life becomes complete. We become whole.

In good health,
VON BRASCHLER
Certified Massage Therapist

Chapter 1

Energy Healing and Healing Hands

Empathy and compassion can help a lot in healing, even compassionate empathy between strangers and different species. You can reach out with healing hands and touch lives in ways that truly make a difference—even if you are a beginner in the art of healing touch.

For many of us, the lives nearest and dearest to our hearts include our pets and plants. Most likely, they do not have medical coverage insurance. They depend on you for all of their immediate needs. The good news is that you can help to heal your pets, your houseplants, and even yourself. It really does not matter how much specialized training you have—just that you put your heart and your hands to good work with the best intentions.

That simple truth was taught to me by a former professor of nursing at New York City University, Dolores Krieger. She once told me a story about finding a lost dog in traffic.

The small dog found itself trapped in the worst traffic imaginable. It squirmed between oncoming cars and darted from side to side, panicked to find itself engulfed in the middle of rush-hour traffic on the notorious New Jersey Turnpike. Drenched and blinded by incessant rain, the ragged dog side-stepped speeding cars and trucks in the never-ending line of bumper-to-bumper traffic.

How the little dog got into this predicament is unknown. People do sometimes abandon unwanted pets on highways as a way of eliminating them from their busy lives. Perhaps that is how this ragged, little dog found itself in the midst of some of the busiest traffic on earth. The New Jersey Turnpike near New York City might be compared to the German Autobahn or the busy streets of Tokyo during rush hour. Crossing the Turnpike is hopeless, a certain death sentence. How long this dog could manage to dodge the endless river of cars in the pouring rain was the only question.

Fortunately, Dolores Krieger and a friend spotted him in the middle of all of this confusion. They pulled their car over to the side, risking their lives to stop traffic long enough to corral the panic-stricken canine. It was a risky gamble that paid off. They grabbed the ragged dog and put him into their car.

Once in the city, the two ladies considered what to do about him. He was shivering, sickly, and shocked by his ordeal. He was so ragged from exposure to the elements that it must have been hard to tell one end of his tangle-haired body from the other. But that is the way shaggy, little dogs sometimes look, especially after hours in the rain.

Dolores Krieger had been working as a waitress at about this time, years before she wrote her groundbreaking book, *The Therapeutic Touch*. Her friend, Dora Van Gelder Kunz, had been trained by noted psychic Charles W. Leadbeater. As a girl with natural psychic abilities, she became the eyes for the elderly clairvoyant, whose own eyes were failing him.

Dora knew what to do for the little dog. Together the two ladies began using their hands to channel healing energy to the dog. This calmed him and stopped his shaking. In time, he recovered completely from the ordeal.

Dora encouraged Dolores to go to college to become a teaching nurse. In time Dolores taught thousands and thousands of nurses and other medical professionals and paraprofessionals how to employ the sort of hands-on healing technique they had used on the little dog. Her students began teaching others and writing books and research papers to add to the great body of books and research that Dolores herself accumulated.

Over the next few years, Dora Kunz began to serve as consultant to hospitals, helping with difficult diagnoses. She taught her amazing healing techniques through the Theosophical Society and continued to involve spiritual healers in such projects as her books, *Spiritual Elements of the Healing Arts* and *Chakras and Human Energy Fields*, which she co-authored with Shafica Karagulla, M.D.

Dora Kunz became the modern bridge for a long line of empathic healers who passed on the tradition of natural folk healing by tutoring others. Kunz had been trained in the Theosophical tradition.

The international Theosophical Society was founded by two spiritually-minded psychics who met in New England more than a hundred years ago. Colonel H. S. Olcott of Civil War fame met Russian psychic Helena Blavatsky at a farmhouse gathering to witness a psychic display. Together the two of them formed the international Theosophical Society in New York City at the turn of the last century. They later moved their headquarters to India for a study of comparative religion and the mysterious powers latent in people.

Colonel Olcott is personally credited with healing thousands in his lifetime and was honored by the government of Ceylon for his selfless works in healing there. He believed that electricity—including bioelectricity—was a latent manifestation of the universal life force that is present and accessible everywhere.

After Olcott came the legendary Theosophical psychic and author C. W. Leadbeater, who trained Dora Kunz. Dora later became national president of the Theosophical Society and to her dying day assisted Dolores Krieger in therapeutic touch workshops throughout the country. Dr. Krieger has extended these workshops around the world and even taught Japanese businessmen how to use energy healing.

Dora Kunz also tutored Dolores Kreiger in meditation. Together they attended psychic healing demonstrations by a traditional folk healer who was visiting the New York area, Colonel Oskar Estebany, a retired Hungarian cavalry officer. There he showed his amazing ability to empathically heal with the touch of his hands.

Years before, Estebany had stunned his neighbors with a display of his awesome ability, healing horses and other barnyard animals with his hands-on technique of focused energy. Many neighbors witnessed his amazing ability to heal simply with the touch of his hands and compassion of his heart. Then one day a neighbor brought a dying child to him, since the nearest doctor was far away. The colonel at first gave his apologies, stating that his healing touch had only been applied to horses and farm animals. But the frantic parent pleaded for him to try. His astounding success made Estebany famous, and he began to demonstrate his technique in barns here and there.

These healing techniques are ancient and universal. Folk healers have employed empathic energy healing throughout the centuries. In different cultures it has different names. It is the oldest form of the healing arts. Healing touch is mentioned in Homer's *Odyssey*. It is also mentioned in ancient Indian Sanskrit texts and depicted in ancient temple reliefs, such as the one at Borobudur in Java, built approximately 800 A.D., which shows the Buddha receiving the healing touch. Perhaps the earliest documented proof of healing touch is found in the Yellow Emperor's *Classic of Internal Medicine*, attributed to Huang Ti, the Yellow Emperor, who died in 2598 B.C. Hippocrates, the Greek physician and father of medicine now associated with the Hippocratic Oath, discussed healing touch as one of his primary therapeutic treatments.

You can employ this natural healing technique to assist your pets. You can use it also to aid the natural healing of your houseplants and other life forms that are near and dear to you. All life is sacred and precious. All life responds to the energy and compassion of the natural healing touch. The technique can be easily learned and employed by anyone with the proper focus and intent. Or as Dolores Krieger has said, everyone can learn to use their hands to help or to heal—even a little dog or a horse in need. It is very natural.

The approach to healing touch that Dr. Krieger taught is a little different from other techniques. The Krieger method, derived from a serious study of Colonel Estebany's success, puts the practitioner's hands in very close proximity to the subject without actually touching. In many similar modalities, touch therapy or healing with your hands involves actual contact. But whether the approach is with Reiki, polarity, yoga healing, Chinese "chi" systems, prana healing, psychic healing, or massage techniques, the results are pretty much the same. The healing touch delivers a rebalanced sense of health and harmony when the intent of the practitioner is to help or to heal. All of these systems involve bodywork in which universal energy all around us and within us can be channeled and directed to balance the energy and life force in another who is near and dear to us. This is as natural and effective as a mother's kiss or hug. Everyone has the potential to use their hands to help or to heal.

Dr. Krieger taught thousands of nurses across the country and throughout the world to use the healing touch in emergency situations. Emergency room nurses code their use of therapeutic touch as "tt" in their medical notes. They use healing touch in ER situations in attempts to stop bleeding, calm patients, and deal with trauma. Of course, this is not done in place of normal emergency room treatment, but in addition to it. Scientific research has demonstrated that healing touch is an effective complementary technique.

I learned the benefits of the healing touch personally when I cut my hand at a workshop in Sioux Falls, South Dakota. I had been leading a small group in Kirlian camera exercises, which measure bioenergy leaving a body that has been stimulated electrically. (The response is measured as an energy burst on a sheet of film paper.) The two-day workshop was almost over, and I was rushing to pack my camera and other things into a box to meet a plane out of town. In my haste, I cut my hand badly on a sheet of glass that I was trying to force into the crowded box.

One of the workshop attendees, a young woman who had driven from out of state to attend, rushed to my side. She grabbed hold of my bleeding hand and placed my other hand on top of it. Then she looked me directly in the eye and told me to center myself and to focus. She placed the thumb of my good hand on top of the bleeding gash and applied gentle pressure. After only a couple of seconds, she told me that it was okay. She turned to walk away, and left the room without looking back.

I lifted my thumb off the cut. It had been a deep, wicked gash, so I was prepared to see the worst. To my surprise, the bleeding had completely stopped, and the wound appeared almost healed. I looked for the helpful woman to thank her, but she had already left the workshop to drive home. There had been no doubt in her mind, it seems, that the healing touch would work for me. And the fact that I had doubts did not seem to impair her efforts.

I could see the amazing power of healing touch with my own eyes. And I could see how people could heal themselves with this technique. After all, I had centered myself, focused, and then placed my own thumb upon the cut to stop the bleeding. I did not even need a bandage.

After this dramatic demonstration, I was eager to learn the healing touch techniques being taught through a hospice program near my home. Nurses associated with the new hospice program had learned the technique at a workshop taught by Dolores Krieger on Orcas Island in Washington State. Dr. Krieger and Dora Kunz taught countless nurses, medical professionals, and paraprofessionals at these workshops around the country; nurses and others who became certified in healing touch in this manner often taught local classes of their own to further spread their knowledge.

I began to attend workshops and eventually met Dr. Krieger herself. I joined a therapeutic touch group and began practicing regularly with other people trained in this technique.

Volunteers at the hospice program found it helpful to use the harmonizing energy of the healing touch to reduce pain and stress in their chronically ill patients. The beauty of the Krieger method for use in hospice care is that practitioners do not actually lay hands upon their patients, who are often extremely sensitive to physical touch.

We would practice these new techniques together for hours until we became quite sensitive to each other's touch. I came to realize that the hand is a double helix and an ideal instrument for sensing energy imbalance in a body. I could see that the human hand is also ideal for delivering energy to correct the gaps and log jams that prevent a body from being whole, balanced, and harmonized.

My own experience in learning to properly heal with my hands involved mainly human subjects. Many of my initial subjects were experienced touch therapy healers themselves, which allowed them to give me accurate feedback.

While I was learning to use my healing hands, I kept thinking about the little dog and the horses of Colonel Estebany who were among the first subjects of these natural healing techniques. Because I love nature so much, it seemed to me that we could be using our healing touch to help the animals and plants around us. Animals and plants do not have medical plans to aid them in their moments of pain and suffering. And they do not have the kind of doubts about healing touch that humans do. Almost every animal mother administers healing touch to her young. It is the only health treatment available to them. Plants and animals live closer to nature than people do. They learn to trust the healing touch instinctively, without what people might call intellectual confusion.

As I became involved with pet massage, and was certified in pet massage therapy, I began to incorporate the healing touch of energy transfer in my routine treatment of animals in addition to massage techniques designed only to rub aching muscles, restore good circulation, and reduce pain to pressure points in the body. The healing touch could aid much more.

Chapter 2

Get Grounded and Focused With Intent and Creative Visualization

To learn how to perform healing touch effectively, it is best to practice on other people first. Ideally, you should practice with other students of this healing art. That way you can provide feedback to each other. Your pets and houseplants cannot provide you with the sort of critique that you will need to begin to perfect your technique.

When you begin to achieve successes that both you and your human subjects can feel and repeat, you will be ready to work with the animals and plants that are dear to you. They will provide a more subtle feedback that you will learn to detect in time.

Learning to heal with your hands obviously requires feeling. You will scan with your hands, assess with your hands, project energy with your hands, and analyze results with your hands. But your hands are not all that is involved. Proper preparation is required as well.

To heal empathically with energized compassion, you must prepare carefully to enter the right state of consciousness. Remember that this is healing art in its purest, most natural expression. The healer, as artist, must enter the correct frame of mind. It matters little what modality of healing touch you wish to follow. Practically all worthwhile forms of hands-on healing by touch therapy have this in common. The healer must prepare to enter a heightened state of awareness.

Hands-on healers should first remove their shoes and sit erect in a chair or on the floor with feet squarely anchored on the ground. A perfect lotus position can be substituted for the erect sitting posture. In such a position, hands-on healers should center themselves by clearing the mind of everything except the healing task ahead. Healers should focus themselves to shut out all external and internal distractions. By their exercise of will, all internal dialogue ceases. Healers then reach the center of their being where the spirit or essential life force resides. In this manner, healers align themselves to tap the life force deep within them and prepare for the energy work ahead.

Healers enter a meditative state of heightened consciousness. By shutting out all external and internal distractions and focusing their attention, healers suspend lower mind functions and begin operating on a higher level. A higher mind becomes superactive in this heightened state of attention.

This heightened state of consciousness enables natural healers to focus energy. The bioenergy that flows naturally through the body is at their command to direct, literally at their fingertips. Once centered, focused, and energized in this state of heightened awareness, the natural healer is ready to approach the subject.

The healer should ask the subject to sit quietly, with shoes removed and feet placed firmly on the ground. The healer should put the subject at ease in a quiet manner without stirring or speaking. The subject may close eyes or keep them open—whatever is most comfortable. Ideally, healing subjects should be centered and focused to receive energy. Asking them to sit quietly and to find a still point deep within themselves encourages them to center themselves and become focused.

This sort of healing is done empathically from spirit to spirit. The spirit of the healer acts empathically to assist the spirit or life force of the healing subject or client. Consequently, the healer will want the subject's physical body to fall asleep, taking with it the body's many physical distractions. Meanwhile, the subject's inner spirit or life essence awakens. As the subject's spirit awakens, the spirit's essential life force becomes more actively awake and energetic. Knowledgeable subjects will center themselves and then slip into meditative consciousness to accomplish this. Other subjects must be coaxed gently to focus and enter a still place deep within, oblivious to outside physical distractions.

The healer works quietly, remaining in a state of heightened attention. The hands of the healer are held just a few inches off the subject's body, as though caressing the surrounding aura. The hands of the healer move from the top of the subject's head down the subject's body, touching the surrounding energy field. The healer's hands move slowly, giving him or her time to assess any impressions that arise from this examination.

This is not so much a physical examination as an examination of the subject's entire essence and life force. The healer might experience a tingling sensation in the hands at certain points during the assessment. At other points, the healer may feel heat in the hands, or even a cold, empty feeling. These odd sensations will give the healer clues regarding the areas of the subject that suffer from imbalance or blockages. These areas should receive extra attention from the healer's sensitive, energized hands.

The healer then directs his or her hands over the subject's body, often working in slow, circular motions. The healer might pause at certain suspect points, all the while focusing on sending energy from the hands to the subject's total body. The healer might feel the subject responding in particular spots to the bioelectrical stimulation of the healing hands by sending back energy. The healer might sense this as a tingling or pulsing, warm feeling in their healing hands. This is an indication that the self-regenerative energy of the subject has been awakened. In a real sense, the healer is "jump-starting" the subject back to a state of self-regeneration or rejuvenation.

Many practitioners of healing touch sense that the ailments of their subjects are due to an imbalance of energy in the body. This concept is expressed in Eastern terminology as the Chinese "chi" and the Indian "prana"—the life force that is believed to flow within the body like a river. This energy flow can become blocked—like a logjam—and the body can become diseased as a result. The perfect balance of body energy is the key to well-being and good health, according to ancient Indian and Chinese health models.

Hindus visualize the energy generated in key regions of the body as swirling vortexes called "chakras," strategically placed in at least seven major points. These chakra energy centers, according to the Hindu model, can wear down like a tired clock and cease to function properly. As a result, energy can cease to flow properly in the part of the body that is governed by that particular chakra. The seven major chakras correspond, incidentally, to the major endocrine glands.

The ancient Chinese health model has a similar view. Chinese medicine maintains that chi runs through the body along meridians, and it is concentrated in strategic parts along the body known as acupressure points. These acupressure points can be accessed to restore balance.

Western allopathic medicine, with its emphasis on treating symptoms more than causes, studies the mechanical movements of muscles lifting bones and nerves carrying impulses with little serious speculations about the root impulse that drives life within the human body. The Eastern model is our best explanation at the moment for the mystery behind the driving force of life. This explanation has proved satisfactory for billions of people in the East for thousands of years and persists to this day.

Energy within the body is a powerful force. The hands-on healer should only put about 15 minutes of energy work into any one session. These energy jolts to the body are not harmful, but they are much more powerful than it might appear on the surface. It is simply not necessary to bombard a weak body with more than 15 minutes of energy work at any one time. The healer can always resume the treatment later in the day or the next day.

Of course, a healer in this focused state of heightened consciousness—oblivious to much of the outside world—might not perceive the passage of time in the normal way. This is particularly true of beginners. In heightened consciousness, people experience a sense of timelessness. The subject, meanwhile, grows heavy and might even begin to fidget after about 15 minutes of energy work by the healer. Uneasiness of the subject provides a cue to the healer that the session has reached a logical conclusion. Otherwise, the healer might compensate by setting a timer, or asking a third person to watch the clock.

Experienced healers will program their sessions during meditation preparation with the conscious intent of only conducting the session for about 15 minutes. With experience, healers develop a feeling for the correct length of a session and can sense when it is time to end. In the state of heightened awareness one acquires a whole new set of senses. This heightened attention will be fully alert in the prepared healer, and will be also activated in the subject during touch therapy, if the subject has been properly centered and focused.

Skeptics often wonder at the conclusion of healing touch whether anything meaningful has happened. Even healers and subjects often wonder whether they can be certain that a session was done properly in a way that should produce results. How can you really know that the session was done properly?

Experienced healers and subjects can answer this question. Both healer and subject can feel the effects of energy work when done properly. The healer clearly feels the energy flowing, and so does the subject. There is no guesswork when healing touch is done properly. The energy is warm and tingly in a way that both parties can feel.

Healing Animals

After practicing for some time on people, the beginning healer acquires a practiced hand for touch therapy and a confidence in procedures that lead to successful results. It is time to begin working with animals.

The animals in our care depend upon us for almost everything. They depend on us for love, shelter, food, emotional support, help, and health care. Because they deserve the very best support, exercise, and care we can provide them, we bring them to professional veterinarians when they are ill. This can never be overlooked in providing proper health care for the animals we love. But as we have seen, healing touch is something that we can give to our loved ones to help restore the energy balance and life force within them, in addition to other care that they might require. Think of healing touch as a booster battery for the ones you love. In providing healing touch, you are aiding their recovery by helping them to rejuvenate themselves.

Of course, you cannot ask your dog, cat, or horse to center itself and find a still, quiet place deep inside. You cannot ask your pet friend to focus its intent and to become quiet. You cannot ask the pet to ground itself by placing its feet firmly on the floor. In short, you cannot verbalize any of the instructions that you would normally impart to human subjects during healing touch to put them into a meditative state of heightened consciousness.

With most animals, you will not need to do any of this, anyway. Animals naturally ground themselves. After all, they are closer to nature than we are. They are close to the earth. Furthermore, animals naturally access the spirit side of their being without shutting down their physical senses. Animals walk with spirit naturally, because they are close to nature. They are sensitive to the unseen world, as many pet owners can attest in recounting psychic abilities of the animals who share their homes. Consequently, they can focus their intent on the healing process.

Animals who receive healing touch naturally become still and quiet. Typically, they do not twitch or blink, but sit quietly through the entire session. They appear to enjoy it and appreciate it immensely. After all, this is similar to the way their own mothers cleaned them and cared for them. Touch is something that animals understand and like very much.

Animals will open their inner spirits to you. They will absorb your energy and bounce energy back to you lovingly. Animals love to share, and love it when you care. Most importantly, they instinctively know how to absorb energy in order to regenerate themselves and restore a healthful balance to their inner life force. That is how animals bounce back so amazingly when they are injured or ill. Because they are so close to nature, they sense how to tap the energy of nature all around them to rejuvenate themselves.

Animals that are unfamiliar with you, of course, might be afraid of the process. That is only because they do not know you and are cautious. Soothing words in a soft voice might woo them. Also, you can communicate with them on a non-verbal level. Your body language helps. Move slowly. Crouch low to the ground, instead of towering over them. You might even put yourself in a prone position, lower your head, or lie on your back near them.

Non-verbal communication with animals can also be telepathic. Many animal behaviorists including Beatrice Leidecker and Penelope Smith have achieved amazing results in teaching people how to communicate with their pets telepathically. That is how animals often communicate with each other. They do not need elaborate language skills. Think about it. Surely you have seen flocks of birds in flight who turn all at once in mid-air. You have watched animals stare at each other face-to-face, and come to a silent understanding. Perhaps all animals, including humans, were once blessed with telepathic ability. Wild animals, including those who share our homes as pets, still have this ability and use it. And animals get along fine without verbal language skills—even between different species. The only question here is whether we can acquire telepathic ability to communicate with them.

Surely it requires practice and patience. And you will want to keep your non-verbal statements simple and positive in ways that animals can accept. As you do for healing, you will want to prepare yourself for telepathic communication. This is easier than you might imagine. Once you have entered a meditative state, you are prepared to communicate telepathically. You will be speaking spirit-to-spirit, after all, apart from the physical world of sound and normal sensory perception. This is extrasensory perception. Focus your intent to communicate telepathically with a certain animal. You must project your will to do this in your new state of heightened awareness.

Do not be surprised when you achieve telepathic communication with an animal. It is hardest, perhaps, with animals you have known for years. Such familiar animals will discount your newfound efforts at unspoken communication, since they have become accustomed to the confusion of your voice, which often conflicts with your body language and your inner thoughts. Animals who know you too well might be reluctant to trust your inner thoughts, since they know your voice and the conflict between your thoughts and your spoken words. Animals just do not understand the inner conflicts in people. It is not surprising that animals do not trust us. People are walking, talking liars by nature. Our words seldom mirror our thoughts and our body language. Other animals, by contrast, have no such inner conflict. Compared to us, they are pure of heart and spirit. If they seem simple, it is because they are not complex and deceptive in the way that people are. In fact, the only animals who attempt to hide their inner feelings are the ones who have lived with people and learned to shield themselves.

While this difference between people and animals might seem sad, consider how gloriously happy your life and the life of your beloved pet can become when you finally do learn to communicate non-verbally. Your pet is fully capable. Are you?

I have a personal story I would like to share about learning to communicate non-verbally with animals. After studying the Leidecker instructional videos and reading the Penelope Smith books on pet communication, I tried to speak telepathically with my own pets. They just looked away. They would not even try to speak with me, it seemed. I considered how they were probably too accustomed to how I communicate with them to try anything new. I decided that I would have better luck with a cat or dog I had never met before.

My chance for that came sooner than I expected. My new gray cat was missing, and I looked for her down an alley. I called, but she did not come. I felt certain that she was somewhere near, so I tried sending out a message to her telepathically.

Little cat, where are you? I tried to project this thought out to her telepathically, wherever she might be.

Then a little black cat appeared out of nowhere. It stood in the alley and stared straight at me.

I took a couple steps closer to the little black cat. It just stood there, staring at me intently.

Then it hit me. My telepathic communication had reached this cat. So I put myself back into the proper state of consciousness to continue my communication.

Where is the little gray cat? I asked.

The black cat blinked. Then it responded with a question: *Little? Gray with a white spot under chin?*

I was puzzled. This cat was asking for details. I was not sure whether the gray cat had a white spot under its chin. Some white spot somewhere, though. That is all I remembered for sure. And my cat was actually no smaller than this one. So the black cat in front of me probably did not consider my cat to be small at all.

Medium sized cat, I answered carefully. *Gray with a little white spot, yes.*

Behind the garage, the black cat responded.

I was not sure that I understood correctly. I seemed to, but I did not trust that I heard correctly. After all, I was hearing for the first time without my ears, and speaking for the first time with a cat on a very mature level.

That garage? I asked, pointing to the right.

The cat simply ran behind the garage. I followed slowly.

As I rounded the corner, I found my gray cat there. It was just as the black cat had told me—even the white spot under its chin. She had one, alright. I really had not noticed before, but the black cat did.

Practice speaking telepathically with your pets. And be patient, because they are not accustomed to trusting non-verbal communication with people. It might even confuse them at first. In time, however, this might work for you.

Healing Plants

You can also use healing touch on your house plants. Energy flows through their living bodies, too. They are subject to imbalances, including energy gaps and blockages. Plants are good at caring for themselves in processing water and light. They extract nutrients from the soil. They even send out roots in search of water and nutrients and extend their vines in search of light. Anything that determined to find life-giving sustenance must have a strong will to survive and a definite consciousness.

I know from work with Kirlian photography that plants respond to electrical stimulation in the same way as people and other life forms—by emitting electrical bursts of their own. The energy burst of a plant bombarded with electrical stimulation looks much the same as the energy burst of a person whose fingertip has been similarly stimulated. We are really not that different in terms of essential life force.

People who have a "green thumb" in working with plants probably exude the healing touch instinctively in their loving attention. Certainly the reverse is just as true with people who exhibit the "purple thumb," killing just about every plant they encounter. The difference is that the green-thumb people display loving empathy for plants. Perhaps, too, they are natural healers who unconsciously perform healing touch.

Consciously performing healing touch on plants will work in the same way it works on animals. As with pets, plants will not require preparation for grounding, centering, or focused intent. Nothing is more grounded than a plant. Plants are also centered—not scattered in their attention, as people tend to be. Furthermore, plants are very focused in their intent, as we can see in their determination to thrive. There is nothing more single-minded and focused than a plant.

The healer, of course, will need to prepare for healing touch by grounding, centering, and focusing intent in a state of heightened consciousness. The healer then assesses the plant and spends approximately 15 minutes running hands alongside it, without actually touching it directly in most cases. The hands should project energy to the plant from a position just a few inches away. The hands should descend along the full length of the plant, including leaves, stems, vines, flowers, and even roots. When the hands are used to assess the energy level of the roots and send new energy to them, you may come into full tactile contact with the pot that surrounds the roots, or with the earth around the plant in the case of plants situated outdoors.

It is helpful to talk soothingly to the plant, and even to attempt telepathic communication. Be advised that plants may be even more simplistic and pure in their expressed thoughts than animals. You will need to really focus your attention to listen to their thoughts and their pain. Plants suffer in silence. They expect so little.

Keep a Journal

As with people and pets, keep a journal of your healing touch sessions with plants. Meditate on the sessions to better understand their significance. Since healing touch is done in a state of heightened consciousness, the healer can best analyze the experience in a similar state. After you meditate on the experience, record the session in your journal. It is best to keep a record of your subjects by date. Record any ailments that they might tell you about. Record your impressions. Record wherever you noted gaps, empty spots, or blockages of energy. Record any place where you might have concentrated your energy work. Note exactly how long you worked, and include your thoughts and schedule for future work.

Chapter 3

Distance Healing, Astral Healing, and Thought Forms

Distance should not discourage you from helping your pets and plants heal. You might find yourself miles away from your loved ones, but the distance should not prevent you from touching them. There are several effective ways to do distance healing. Just as we assist healing with energy at our fingertips, we can employ energy for healing over great distances. Energy is boundless. It does not observe maps or street barriers. Once focused and directed properly, energy moves from one point to another affecting change. In a sense, this use of energy to affect change is magic. You become the agent of change. And this sort of change is only natural, based on the elements and dynamic principles of nature.

You can utilize the energy inside you and all around you in many helpful ways. Your healing energy can be directed with focused intent to targets miles away. If you enter a state of heightened consciousness with meditation, you can even leave your physical body for astral travel and astral healing. You can load your healing energy into a receptacle, such as a crystal, and send it to a loved one. You can direct your healing energy in chants that you personalize for your loved ones. All of these distance healing techniques work in much the same way that healing touch works—through the personal transmission of healing energy that is directed with focused intent.

Let us first consider the techniques and benefits of distance healing with thought forms:

Healing with Thought Forms

Our thoughts can be powerful. We can give them form and substance and project them outside ourselves like arrows to a target or signals to a receiver. In doing so, we energize and drive them with the full force of our focused intent. We shape them with the intense inner magical power of transformation called creative visualization. Whatever we conceive and perceive, we can achieve.

Thought forms can take many shapes. They can take the shape of healing, with specific applications in mind. They can include a particular subject as recipient of these healing signals. They can focus on a particular recipient in a particular location. As agents of change with the amazing magical ability of creative visualization, we can do all of that with pinpoint precision. Whether the subject of our healing signal is trapped somewhere in a tunnel out of sight or floating somewhere in a plane lost in the clouds, we can always direct this healing signal precisely to the target recipient. That is because we have something better than radar or sonar. We can visualize our loved ones in our mind's eye and always find them in that way. As a result, our arrows always find their marks. This is real magic. It is electromagnetic attraction. It is karma on a basic level—the karma of attraction. When you feel something for someone deeply, you are always connected with that person and can find them in any crowd.

Thought forms that you empower with the full force of your focused intent and your will to drive them assume an added dimension as forces in the universe. These charged thought forms become thought power. And power can do many wonderful things, if applied in the right way where needed. Power can restore life, rejuvenate, and transform. In the case of human beings who generate thought power, we are talking about essential life energy force. Such life force dwells deep within us at the seat of our soul essence, our spirit. When this life force totally leaves us, our physical life ends. When we share some of this life force with others, it restores life. This is the divine spark of life that resides within each of us as a great gift. The beauty is that this gift can be shared.

Astral Healing

When you enter a meditative state of heightened consciousness with focused intent, it is possible to leave your physical body in astral travel to help heal a distant friend. In a state of heightened awareness, almost anything is possible. The trick is to leave your physical body in a safe place, while your astral double leaves on a trip of its own.

Astral travel can take you anywhere you want to go. You only need to visualize the place or individual that you wish to see, and then desire to be there. If you focus your intent in this manner and drive your intent with the full power of your will, you can go virtually anywhere. Your spirit is not limited by the physical world. It is at home everywhere and moves freely outside the limited laws of physics.

One advantage to healing during astral travel over healing with energized thought forms is that astral travel allows you to personally inspect the subject whom you are visiting. You can see and feel the needs of this ailing friend. It does not matter that you leave your physical body without eyes, ears, fingertips, nose, and a tongue. In a state of heightened consciousness, your astral double has even greater perception.

Astral bodies are very different from physical bodies. They are pure spirit and energy. In your astral body, you can reach into someone and touch them very deeply. You are not reaching with hands and tearing through flesh to do this. You are melding your pure energy with the vital life forces deep inside another. You are reaching inside and unblocking energy clogs, restoring balance, and setting chakras back to proper working order. You are touching spirit-to-spirit without physical barriers. This is perfectly safe and perfectly effective.

I have personally witnessed how thought forms and also astral travel have power to heal at a distance. Like others, I was a bit of a skeptic at first. A mystic always wants to experience something fully and personally before attaching belief to any sort of knowledge. Reading about something might inspire a person, but it does not convince a mystic in the same way personal experience does. My personal experience involved a little cat named Miss Ben.

Miss Ben, the Miracle Cat

Miss Ben was a little tonkanese cat that I rescued from a basement. Her alcoholic owner, who truly loved her, would rub her the wrong way whenever he tried to pet her after too many drinks. Cats are sensitive and do not like being mauled, even accidentally. The lovable drunk named his (female) cat Ben, and the odd name stuck. If the cat tried to get away from him, he would bang her against the wall or hold her under the shower to discipline her. Miss Ben tried to climb out the basement windows, but only succeeding in leaving claw marks everywhere along the shuttered window ledge.

I rescued Miss Ben and gave her occasional freedom to play outdoors. All she really wanted was to be free and breathe fresh air. One day, poor Miss Ben was hit by a car. I was horrified. She was crippled in two places and unable to walk. In fact, her veterinarian said that the severity of the double fractures made them inoperable in all likelihood, unless I considered taking her to a hospital back East or requesting the local university to attempt it. Most likely, he said, Miss Ben would need to be etherized.

The doctor said to watch her carefully for a week and then bring her back for another examination. After a week, he might be willing to recommend her to the local university staff for corrective surgery. That week looked pretty long and grueling to me, particularly since I was scheduled to make a business trip to London that could not be postponed. Poor Ben lay in a cardboard box with the front cut away, so that she could occasionally drag her limp body to nearby water, food, and litter.

I asked my neighbor and her fiancé to watch Miss Ben for me, and to take her to the veterinarian with any changes in her tender condition. They visited Ben twice a day to clean her litter box, provide fresh nourishment, and give her love and comfort. It is about all that anybody could do, we thought.

Far away in London in a strange hotel room, I felt unable to help her, and sad that I had abandoned her during her darkest hour. Then an inspiration came upon me. I was not powerless, despite the distance. I could visualize her clearly in my mind's eye during meditation and then send my healing thought forms to her.

I did this for the first two nights away, but I was still worried because I could not see her. So I decided to leave my body and visit her in astral travel. It was the first time that I had ever tried to visit somebody in my astral body for healing, and I was amazed how clear everything appeared to me. I meditated until I reached a state of heightened consciousness and felt complete detachment from my physical body. I entered this state with the intent to leave my body and travel back to my house across the ocean. I held a picture of my sick cat in my mind's eye, as I slipped out of normal consciousness. I engaged the full force of my will, as projected from my lower abdomen, to drive my intent forward.

I found myself almost instantly in my bedroom back across the ocean. I was positioned in front of my crippled little cat. She lay limp in the cutaway cardboard box, with little food or water taken. I began to project my astral body into the area of her broken leg and tail bone. I concentrated on infusing her with energy and melding her together, not knowing exactly how the bones should be fused. She seemed to react to my presence, or my energy input, but did not recognize me as being in the room in any way.

The next few nights, I went across the ocean to her in the same manner and infused energy into her limp body. I concentrated on healing the broken bones and melding them together. With my astral body, I could reach into her easily and do this. Each night, she seemed to respond more and more to my presence. On the last night she seemed to recognize me and reached out to greet me in a way she had never done before. She inched forward, with less discomfort than I remembered her showing, and licked at me. It was like the way a kitten and its mother relate to each other's intimacy in grooming. She seemed happy to see me—and she really did see me! I am certain of this.

The next night when I visited her, I did not find her in her cutaway box. She was nowhere in the room. I started to fear the worst, but then a quiet comfort came over me. Somehow, I knew that she was alright.

The next day I came home from London. I rushed to the bedroom. Miss Ben was there and responded to me warmly. She bolted out of her box and rushed forward to lick my nose with great joy. She seemed very happy to see me and affectionate toward me in a way I had never seen before, except in our recent astral meeting. It was as though she recognized me from my astral visit.

My neighbor was there in the room. She explained that Ben had been to the doctor's office the previous day for her scheduled follow-up visit. What the doctor found was truly amazing. Miss Ben was fully recovered and showed no sign of any broken bones. She did not need an operation or any further treatment. In fact, he was so surprised at her miraculous and sudden recovery that he questioned whether it was the same cat. Well, there is only one little Miss Ben, of course.

Miss Ben today climbs trees as well as any of our neighborhood squirrels, often outmaneuvering them in playful romps through the branches.

She shows no signs of the badly broken bones that once crippled her. Well, that is not exactly true—one bone fits together oddly. I attribute that to the fact that neither Ben nor I knew anything about cat anatomy at the time we did the energy work to help her heal. Even so, Miss Ben shows no discomfort and romps with the best of them now, a totally free and healthy little cat.

Loading Energy Objects

It is possible to load healing energy into objects, such as crystals, that you can send to sick friends. The recipient should hold the stone tightly in one hand and meditate to fully appreciate the benefit of the healing vibrations that have been stored for them. In the case of a pet or a plant, the stone should be positioned next to them.

Vibrational messages can be stored in virtually anything. That is how psychic investigators are able to use articles of clothing or other personal objects to pick up signals left by the person who handled that object. Such objects can contain emotional sensations, such as fear or anger. They can also contain specific signals that were consciously loaded into the object.

Quartz crystals are ideal for storing vibrational information for many reasons. They can trap a signal within their many facets until someone releases it. Such crystals can also be used to transmit, amplify, and focus a signal. That is why large quartz crystals have been used for years as recorders. Of course, a person could store information in another stone or object.

The process is really very simple: The sender holds the object tightly in the right hand and sends the information as a vibrational signal or energy wave into the object. In the case of a healing stone, the sender as healer visualizes the intended subject or recipient of healing energy. That energy wave is then stored in the object until it is unlocked by the intended recipient. Since the energy was intended for a specific recipient through use of visualization and focused intent, the energy waits for that person to release.

This is a form of very focused, personal communication. The stored signal is a communications delivery mechanism, like a telephone or radio.

I used to exchange healing stones with a group of like-minded friends in Oregon. We would send these stones through the mail to each other, loading them with the healing energy and emotional support that we thought was needed at that particular time in each other's lives. It did not matter that we no longer lived together in the same woods in Oregon, as we had previously. We could still help each other heal by sending healing stones back and forth.

It works the same way with our pets and plants. If the healing stone (or other energy receptacle) is simply put next to the pet or plant, the energy will be imparted. It is best, of course, if the stone comes into physical contact with the subject. You might put the stone squarely against the plant, so they are touching. Or you might put the stone next to your dog or cat as it sleeps in its bed. The healing energy will find its mark.

Chapter 4

Chakra Healing and Chi

Chakra healing is another effective method that you can perform on your pets and plants. Pets have chakras or energy centers in their bodies just like people. In fact, most pets are mammals, and thus very similar to humans in their makeup. There may be minor differences, as we will discover, but very few of any consequence.

Similarly, plants have energy meridians and key access points for the energy that runs through their limbs. Kirlian photography proves that plants generate energy in bursts very similar to those of animals. Research on plants by noted polygraph expert Cleve Backster and others demonstrates convincingly that plants are sensitive bundles of energy and respond to electrical stimuli, much the way people do. Energy healing that focuses on key centers or meridians, therefore, works just as well on plants as on people.

Chakra healing and acupressure are time-tested and proven techniques for rebalancing the overall energy flow in a living body by concentrating on key energy centers. There are various ways to perform chakra healing or its Chinese counterpart. The empathic healer can use healing hands to stimulate energy flow at key centers in the body. The empathic healer can lay healing stones on or near energy centers. Another technique involves astral healing in which the empathic healing treats the subject while in an astral body.

These techniques have been used effectively in the East for thousands of years and can be adapted for pets and plants. All life forms from fauna to flora are pretty much the same—energy beings encapsulated in physical bodies. The metaphysical view of the mystic is that all life is comprised of the same essential life force that is manifest on this physical plane as electromagnetic energy. The Kirlians called it bioplasma. Others might call it psychic energy, life essence, or spirit. Whatever you choose to call it, it is one and the same for all of us. Energy within and around us sustains us when we have enough of it in proper balance flowing properly through us.

Healing Hands

Let us first consider stimulating energy centers in the bodies of our pets and plants with our healing hands. Healing touch is easy to do, as we have seen. The empathic healer simply enters a state of heightened consciousness and then scans the subject from top to bottom for anomalies or aberrations in the flow of energy. The healer should not begin until the hands feel sensitive and ready. For most people, the hands begin to tingle or feel warm when they reach a state of heightened awareness and focused intent. When ready, the healer extends his or her hands a few inches from either side of the body. The healer will normally feel gaps or blockages in the flow of energy as warm spots, cold spots, or spots that make the healer's hands pulsate or tingle. After the healer has assessed the condition with this scan, he or she will run hands over the body again, slowly beginning at the head and working down to the bottom. Once the bottom is reached, the healer will start again from the head, usually keeping his or her hands a few inches off the body of the subject, unless it feels appropriate to pause in a certain spot and actually make tactile contact.

In working through the whole body in this fashion, the empathic healer pauses at cold spots, hot spots, empty spots, or tingling spots that would suggest energy blocks or gaps. I remember spending several minutes on the leg of a human subject at a workshop in Sioux Falls, South Dakota. I sensed a coldness and emptiness there that suggested no energy whatsoever in that leg. Outwardly, this leg looked just the same as his other one. But no matter how hard I tried sending energy to this cold, empty leg, I could sense no change. Then somebody laughed, and the man lifted up his blue jeans to reveal a wooden leg underneath. That pretty well proved to everyone in the workshop that the bounce-back technique of sensing energy flow through the living body really works. His artificial leg, of course, had no energy running through it, but was hollow and cold in the same way that I had sensed it empathically.

When you use your healing hands on energy centers in the living body, you naturally want to focus on those key centers where they appear. Work your hands over these energy centers, either pausing or rotating your hands in small, clockwise circles over them for about a minute. Personally, I prefer the circular motions. The Tellington system works much this way, and so do Hindu *mudras*, or hand gestures. (Hand gestures are also used in Chinese healing.) You must do what feels right, as you develop sensitivity with experience.

As you move your healing hands over your subject, remember that your hand movements direct the energy that is all around us and inside us all. That directed energy, set in motion by our healing intent, can move things, transform things, and affect things in a positive, healing way.

I prefer to make circular motions directly over the chakras because it helps me set them back into proper motion. In the Indian system, the proper motion of these vortexes is clockwise. As I work, I visualize setting these internal "clocks" back into proper working order.

The same holds true when you use the Chinese model, in which acupressure points serve as key access spots for the meridians that carry energy through the body. The healer can employ healing touch to stimulate the meridian lines, concentrating on acupressure points.

The chakra locations in most mammalian pets are much the same as with people, with some notable differences. There are seven major chakras in dogs, cats, and horses—just as there are seven major chakras in people. (Please refer to illustrations.) The root chakra is located at the base of the tail. The sacral chakra is located between the hips and over the spine. The solar plexus chakra is located in the middle of the back at the rib cage base. (This is where ribs meet at T10, the tenth thoracic vertebra.) The heart chakra is located in the middle of the sternum (in the concave center of the chest at the base of the neck). The throat chakra is located between the scapulas at C7, the seventh cervical vertebra. The brow chakra is located above the eyes on the forehead. The crown chakra is located on the top of the head between the ears.

Since the root, sacral, solar plexus, and throat chakras on these pets are all located on their backs and along the spine, it is best to position your hands along their spines and backs. You will need to put your healing hands under the neck and directly on the chest, however, to access the heart chakra of your dog, horse, or cat. You can best access the brow chakra on your dog, cat, or horse on the forehead, and their crown chakra directly on top of the head.

The root chakra governs the spinal column, kidneys, stress responses, feet, and legs. Is is associated with the adrenal gland, the psychological function of survival, and the purpose of survival or will to live. It is often seen as red.

The sacral chakra governs the reproductive system and lower abdomen. It is associated with the gonads, desire, pleasure, and the will to feel emotions. It is often seen as orange.

The solar plexus chakra governs the stomach, liver, gall bladder, and upper abdomen. It is associated with the pancreas, laughter, anger, and the power of the will. It is often seen as yellow.

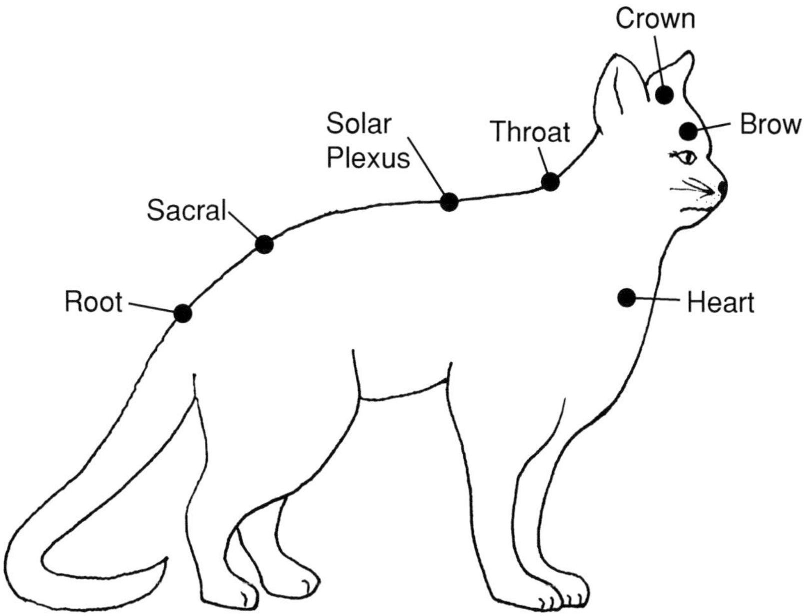

Chakra System in Cats and Dogs

The chakra system placement in animals is the same as in people. There are seven major energy centers within the chakra system.

1. **Root**—Located at the base of the tail
2. **Sacral**—Located between the hips over the spine
3. **Solar plexus** Located in the middle of the back at the rib cage base
4. **Heart**—Located in the middle of the sternum
5. **Throat**—Located between the scapulas
6. **Brow**—Located above the eyes on the forehead
7. **Crown**—Located on top of the head between the ears

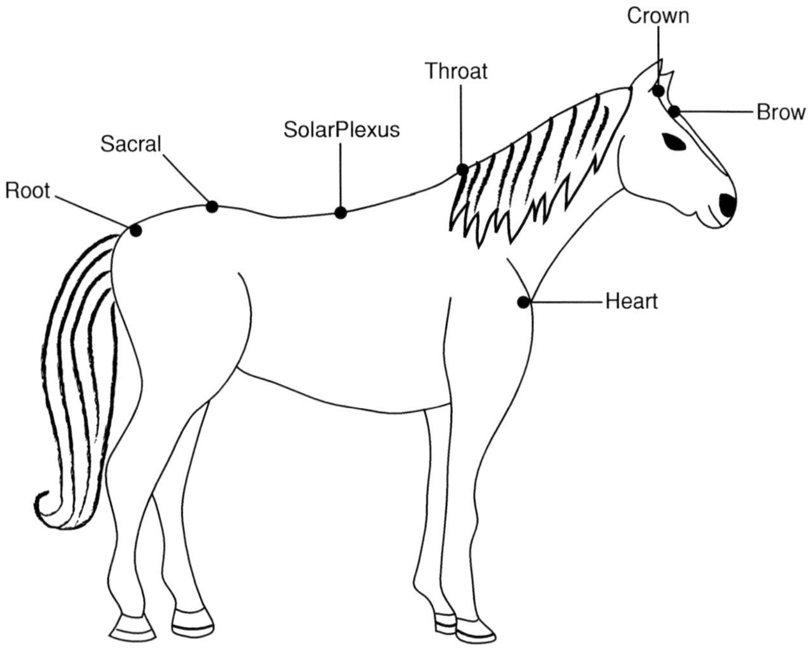

Chakra System in Horses

The heart chakra governs the heart, circulatory system, arms, chest, and hands. It is associated with the thymus, loving, balance, transformation, and the color green.

The throat chakra governs the bronchial tubes, vocal cords, lungs, ears, and respiratory system. It is associated with the parathyroid and thyroid, grieving, communication, expressiveness, higher emotions, and the color blue.

The brow chakra governs the lower mind, eyes, nose, and nervous system. It is associated with the pituitary gland, dreaming, intuition, imagination, visionary thinking, compassion, wisdom, the personality, and the color indigo.

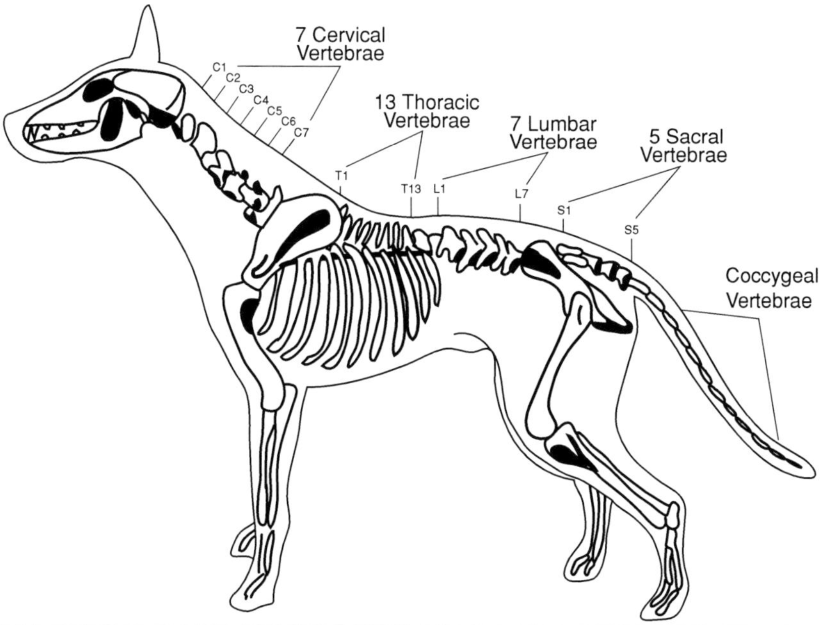

Vertebrae System in Dogs

The crown chakra governs the higher mind. It is associated with the pineal gland, bliss, understanding, holism, higher knowledge, the soul, and the color violet.

Traditional Chinese Acupressure

In the Chinese health system, main indications in our dogs and cats suggest which acupressure point along the energy meridians in the body need attention.

Shock or sunstroke in your dog or cat suggests *yen hong*, an acupressure point located at the upper third of the phylum. These indications also suggest that you access *wei jian*, an acupressure point located at the tail at the point between the last sacral and caudal 1.

Cold or shock could suggest accessing *shan gen*, an acupressure point located at the middle of the nose.

Spasm, colic, sunstroke, or shock could suggest *er jian*, an acupressure point located between the spinous process of C7 (the seventh cervical vertebra) and T1 (the first thoracic vertebra).

Fever, lower body temperature, and traumatic inflammation suggest *da zhui*, an acupressure point located between the spinous process of C7 and T1.

Shoulder sprain, forearm sprain, and fever suggest *yao dao*, an acupressure point located between T1 (the first thoracic vertebra) and T2 (the second thoracic vertebra).

Pain and shoulder sprain suggest *chen zhu*, an acupressure point located between T3 and T4.

Loin sprain and rheumatism suggest *xaun shu*, an acupressure point located between T13 (the thirteenth thoracic vertebra) and L1 (the first lumbar vertebra).

Sciatica indicates that you access *bai hui*, located between L7 (seventh lumbar vertebra) and S1 (first sacral vertebra).

Paralysis of the tail and rheumatism of the loins indicates *wei ben*, an acupressure point located on the blood vessel in the middle of lower surface of the tail.

Sprain or paralysis of digits suggests that you access *liu feng*, an acupressure point located between toes and at the skin folds at the three joints of each leg.

Arthritis of hip bones or sprain indicates *saen tang*, an acupressure point located on the saphenous vein on the inner surface of the thigh.

Obviously, the empathic healer would be wise to gain an understanding of animal anatomy before attempting to access Chinese acupressure points, although a sensitive healer will acquire a natural feeling for where they are located. This can be done while working unobtrusively on the subject's body to scan and access the subject's energy field. (Please refer to illustration and chart.)

Chart 1
Traditional Acupressure Point for the Dog and Cat

Point	Location	Main Indication
#1 Yen Hong	Upper one-third of philum	Shock, sunstroke
#2 Shan gen	Middle of nose	Shock, cold
#9 Er jian	Apex of convex surface of auricula, bilateral	Shock, spasm, colic, sunstroke
#12 Da zhui	Between spinous process of C7 & T1, one point	Fever, traumatic inflammation, lower body temp.
#13 Yao dao	Between T1-T2, one point	Sprain of shoulder and forelimb, fever
#14 Chen zhu	Between T3-T4, one point	Pain, sprain of shoulder
#18 Xaun shu	Between T13-L1, one point	Sprain of loin, rheumatism
#19 Ming men	Between L2-L3, one point	Sprain of loin, rheumatism
#22 Bai hui	Between L7-S (K)1, one point	Sciatica
#26 Wei jian	Attic of tail, one point (Last sacral, caudal 1)	Shock, sunstroke
#28 Wei ben	On blood vessel in the middle of lower surface of the tail, one point	Paralysis of tail, rheumatism of loin
#62 Liu feng	Between toes at skin fold, three points each leg	Sprain and paralysis of digits
#72 Saen tang	On spahenous vein on inner surface of thigh, bilateral	Arthritis of hip bones, sprain

In Chinese tradition, physical contact is made with these acupressure points. It is also possible to access these key energy points without making tactile contact through healing touch done inches away from the body surface. The healer's energy is sent through the fingertips to a spot on the subject's body where the healer points. In this fashion, the healer directs or draws out energy at the acupressure point. Since the principle at work here is actually electromagnetism, the hands can send or receive energy in this fashion without making tactile contact with the subject's physical body.

Acupressure points on your houseplants are not really that hard to find. Look for joints between stems and leaves, where the new leaves begin to extend from the stems. Look for the joints between leaves and flowers. Then look for the joints on the stem of the houseplant itself. Everywhere a new growth extends from a previous growth, key energy centers are present. Find these connecting joints to access the natural acupressure points within your houseplant. The same holds true for outdoor plants and trees.

Reflex Points

The ears of dogs, cats, and horses contain sensitive reflex points that you can trigger with gentle thumb pressure to affect other parts of their bodies. People sometimes refer to these as acupuncture points if they work them with precision healing needles, or acupressure points if they work them with gentle fingertip pressure. I prefer to cradle the ear in my two hands and apply gentle downward pressure to these reflex points in the ear with one thumb.

It becomes obvious when you work these reflex points in the ear that energy is being triggered at certain parts of the body and that the points are directly connected to these remote parts of the body.

Dogs are especially appreciative and cooperative with therapy work centered on the ears. Dogs generally love gentle handling of their ears or areas around them. Horses also are generally cooperative and appreciative of this sort of energy therapy on the ear reflex points. Cats can be temperamental and slow to accept this sort of treatment, as they generally do not like anybody to touch their ears. Nonetheless, this sort of therapy works well on cats, too, when you introduce them to it slowly. You might start by simply stroking the ears on the outside to begin with, then advance to internal stroking, and eventually to therapy work on the ear's reflex points. It might take you several days to work up to actually triggering the ear reflex points.

Please refer to the chart marked "Ear Reflex Points" to see location of these points on the ears and the area that each reflex point affects throughout the body.

Sensitive reflex points on the paws of cats and dogs can be triggered in the same manner to affect the flow of healing energy to remote locations throughout the body. The approach is the same as with the ear reflex points. Acupressure can be applied to these points with the fingertips or thumb. (Acupuncturists, who are professionally trained in the art of accessing energy points in the body with needles, also work these points in the paws of cats and dogs). Again, I prefer to cradle the paw of the dog or cat in both hands and apply gentle downward pressure with one thumb at the designated points. Think of the weight of a nickel in your hand as you apply very gentle pressure to the animals. Work slowly, gently, and patiently.

Please refer to the illustration marked "Paw Reflex Points" for a guide to the various pressure points in the paws of your dog or cat and the corresponding locations these points trigger.

Laying on Healing Stones

It is difficult to lay healing stones over chakra centers when your subject is a houseplant, a fidgeting puppy, or a cat. Gradually, however, your pet can become comfortable with you and these healing sessions. This type

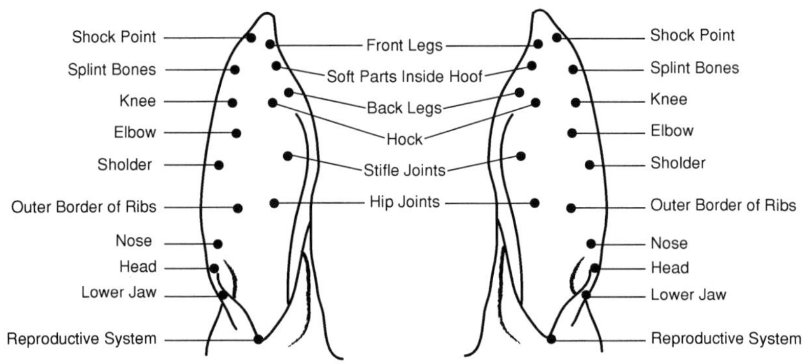

Ear Reflex Points
(Dog, Cat, or Horse)

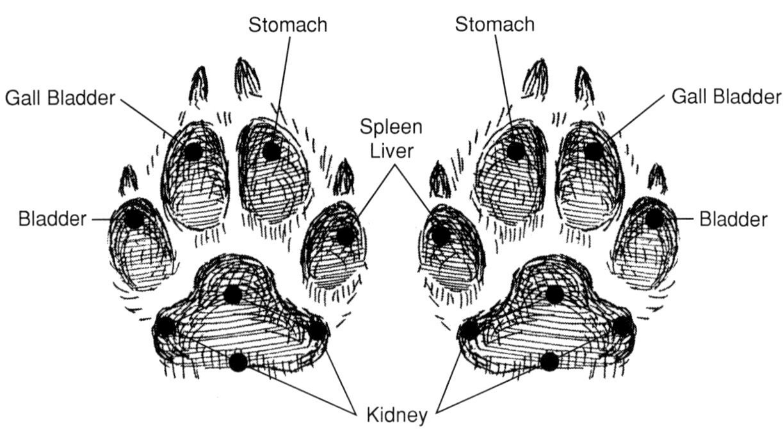

Paw Reflex Points
(Dog or Cat)
The Paws—Hindlimb

of natural healing is soothing to the touch and generally leaves the subject feeling balanced and whole again.

In the beginning, it might be better for you to hold healing stones that are associated with certain energy centers to that particular part of your pet's body. If you sense that more than one chakra in your pet needs energy healing, you can work with one stone and then another, as you work your way from one chakra to the next. In that way, you will slowly but surely accomplish chakra energy balancing in your pet.

Holding a healing stone to the subject also works for houseplants. With most plants, it is practically impossible to lay various healing stones across their bodies. Their bodies rise vertically from the ground and cannot be weighted down with stones in most cases. Also, it is difficult to determine where their energy centers are located, other than near joints between leaves and stems and joints between leaves and flowers. You could either hold a healing stone to the plant or simply lay the stone near the plant.

Various healing stones are traditionally believed to have properties to energize various energy centers in the body of animals. Some of this information is based on solid folklore of traditional folk healers who have established a working relationship with various stones. Some of this is based on the color of the stone to match the energetic color of the chakra or energy center. Different colors vibrate at different levels, indicating a different type of energy wave in each color. Stones all vibrate at different levels, too, based on their colors and properties of their signature energy waves. Consequently, certain stones relate to various parts of the body. They vibrate at similar rates. In this way, a healing stone that is associated in color and energy frequency with a certain energy center in the body restores the harmonic resonance of that part of the body by restoring the energy frequency that resides there. Harmonic resonance strengthens the body and establishes well-being. The energy is once again balanced, and the subject is made whole.

In addition to specific healing gemstones of various colors, you can effectively substitute clear quartz crystal for any healing stone. Quartz crystal exhibits white light, which contains the other colors within it. Also, you can program a quartz crystal to assume the healing vibrations of any color by holding it tightly in the palm of your right hand and meditating with focused intent on the chosen color. In this way, you transfer the color energy you have generated by your creative visualization with focused intent into the stone. This is true magic, and it works every time when done properly.

Clear quartz crystals in the palm of your right hand can also be directed over the body from one energy center to another. This is true even when healing stones are positioned over the energy centers. The crystal amplifies the energy from your hand, transforms it, and focuses it. Of course, you could also effectively use your hands to focus your energy on each energy center and move from one energy center to the next.

Double terminated quartz crystals are ideal for drawing negative energy or energy blocks from the body, when the purpose is not to put energy into the body but draw certain types of energy out of it.

With regard to the seven major chakras that horses, dogs, and cats share with you, consider this list of stones from traditional folk healing:

First chakra: Popular healing stones include bloodstone, garnet, smoky quartz, obsidian, black onyx, and rhodonite,

Second chakra: Popular healing stones include ruby, garnet, citrine, amber, and carnelian.

Third chakra: Popular healing stones include yellow citrine, topaz, sulphur, calcite, apatite, and malachite.

Fourth chakra: Popular healing stones include aventurine, green tourmaline, emerald, pink tourmaline, rose quartz, malachite, and periodot.

Fifth chakra: Popular healing stones include turquoise, aquamarine, gem-silica, amazonite, chrysoscholla, and celestite.

Sixth chakra: Popular healing stones include sodolite, lapis, amethyst, fluorite, azurite, and sapphire.

Seventh chakra: Popular healing stones include clear quartz, diamond, selenite, gold topaz, and heloidor.

As you can see, other colors beyond the seven major chakra colors have become associated with the chakras. Black has become associated with the first or lower chakra, in addition to deep red. Red has become associated with the second chakra, in addition to orange. And orange has become associated with the third chakra, in addition to its dominant color, yellow. Pink has become associated with the fourth or heart chakra, in addition to green, its major color. The sixth chakra is sometimes seen in violet, in addition to its main color, indigo. Meanwhile, the crown or seventh chakra is seen in gold and white, in addition to violet. This is because the colors of the chakras blend to a degree, like the colors in a light spectrum. It is sometimes hard to tell where one color in the light spectrum ends and the next begins. We are all light beings, including our pets and our plants, and we exhibit the energy of all of the light colors within us.

You can program a large generator crystal to project precisely the healing energy that is needed by your pet or plant, and then position it next to your loved one. This is particularly good for plants, since the large healing crystal is just as stationary as a plant. Both are grounded in their positions. A large crystal in such a stationary position, however, can generate an amazing amount of energy once you program it with the proper focused intent.

One last word about healing stones: You should monitor the effect of these stones on your plants or pets and not overexpose your loved ones to their dynamic quality for too long a period. A few minutes at a time should be enough. Watch for signs of exhaustion or tension that may indicate that the healing stones have worked their wonders long enough.

Astral Healing

Astral healing, as we have seen previously, is healing in your astral body outside of your physical body. This is truly a case of the emotional body of the healer seeking to impact the energetic level of the emotional body of the subject. The astral body, then, is the emotional body, as well as the etheric double. When we become ill, this illness often occurs first on the emotional or etheric level, with the energy of this level impacting the physical level that is immediately below it.

When we ground and center ourselves to leave our bodies in a focused state of heightened awareness with the intent to heal, we travel in an astral body that is roughly a double of the physical body. This astral body is a little larger than the more compact and dense physical body that it superimposes itself upon as an outer energy shell. The astral body does not have eyes, ears, or nose. Consequently, it learns to function through practice with another kind of perception—higher awareness. It senses and feels in a different way that becomes acute and effective with experience. The astral body is not physically apparent to the subject in most cases. But we must consider that our pets are keenly aware and psychic and often can see into the spirit world around them. Our plants also function normally without eyes and ears, relaying on an awareness that people do not normally experience. So your presence as an astral healer will be noticed by your subjects, when you enter your astral body to heal your pets or plants. But they will become comfortable with you. Be ready, however, for younger dogs and cats to "freak out" at first when you approach them in this manner. This will pass quickly, since animals are more psychic than people as a rule. Also, your pets will recognize you by feel. Your presence will be familiar to them.

In attempting to reactivate ailing chakras or energy centers in the body of your pets and plants, you must begin to function differently as a healer in your astral body than you have ever functioned before. You must forget the limitations of the physical world and begin operating as a spirit wrapped in energy. In fact, you are pure energy in this form.

You can reach right into the body of your plant or pet in astral form and actually touch the energy centers that need help. You can put them into motion again just as easily as you would wind up a worn-down clock. But you must be in a meditative state and leave your physical body to do this. This is not sleepwalking or trance possession. Nor is it hypnotic behavior. Your physical body must be safely tucked away in a corner, remaining in a meditative state.

You will know for certain that your astral body has left your physical body when you first begin to hover above the room, looking down at your physical self in a meditative state. When you actually succeed in leaving your body consciously, you will feel a sort of snap at the instant of separation. Then you will find yourself floating aimlessly at first in an etheric state. Your first task will be to learn to move directly in such an astral body. You do this by projecting yourself to a specific location by thought. You now are operating with a higher consciousness, where your creative visualization is instantly empowered. You think of where you want to go and project yourself there with your thoughts. You need to focus your attention and your intent on where you want to go and what you want to do.

Astral healing can be done anywhere and at anytime. There are no physical limitations. There is no physical touch. There is only pure energy healing, which you do in a spirit body. You must practice leaving your body and projecting yourself with focused intent and awareness before you can seriously attempt to heal any beloved pet or plant in this manner. When you are ready, this might become the most powerful and effective form of healing that you can offer to your loved ones.

Chapter 5

Gentle Stroking or Massage

As a pet massage therapist, I can assure you that gentle stroking has a very positive therapeutic value for your pet, and even for your plants. Massage is widely recognized for stimulating circulation, reducing swelling, and reducing tension in people. It is also acclaimed for relaxing muscles, warming muscles prior to use, easing muscle spasms, increasing range of motion, and breaking down adhesions. At times, the healing touch of massage feels like magic.

Pets will respond to massage even better than people do, as amazing as that might sound. Remember that your pet is accustomed to its mother's gentle stroking. Many pets groom each other as a sign of friendship or affection. Because your pet will find gentle stroking to be natural and non-threatening, you should have no trouble keeping your pet in position for you to perform massage. Most pets, in fact, will not squirm that much—young animals and newcomers to massage being the possible exceptions. If you go slowly and use gentle strokes and moves that do not startle your pet, even young dogs and anxious kittens should settle down in time (although some animals might be too young for massage, and really do not need it).

What makes massage on your dog, horse, or cat even easier is that you can use many of the same basic massage strokes or moves that have been proven to work on people. All mammals have a lot in common, of course, even if some of us walk on only two of our limbs. Consequently, you might want to review a book on massage techniques and adapt them for your pets, realizing that you need to go very gently and slowly.

The basic massage techniques that I'm going to introduce in this book for your four-legged friends are simple Swedish, essalen, sports therapy, and myofascial release techniques. There are many more good massage and physical therapy maneuvers that you could apply; however, the basic techniques in this book will give you a good starting point. These are techniques that I have been trained to use on animals, and I use them myself as a massage therapist.

Assessment

Observe your pet as it stands in front of you to determine whether its hips seem cocked to one side or its legs seem abnormally extended. If you have somebody with you who could assist, have that person walk the animal toward you and away from you two or three times to determine whether the animal is walking normally or displays cocked hips and uneven strides to compensate for basic imbalance in posture. Such imbalance could suggest range of motion therapy. Note what you observe on a sheet that includes the name of the animal, its age, and medical history.

Introduction

After you have removed your jewelry and anything worn by your pet (including a collar), greet the pet and gently introduce it to a session of hands-on massage. Do this by approaching carefully with a sort of hug from the back. That is, once the animal sees you and becomes comfortable with your presence, begin the massage session by approaching the animal from the back with your hands placed gently on both sides of its head or one hand on its head in a comforting fashion. Do not be concerned whether the animal is sitting or reclining, as long as it is comfortable and relatively still.

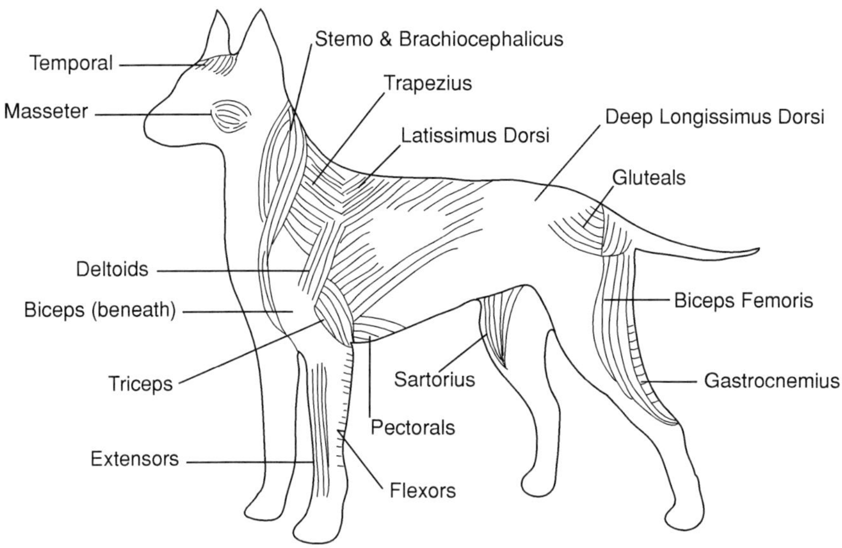

Dog Anatomy: The Muscular System

With a dog or cat, it will probably be best to work on a table or even on the ground, which should be covered by a blanket or heavy towel to keep the animal warm and cozy.

The Head

Gently begin rubbing the area around the head and ears with your finger pads in small circular motions. Do not apply more than a nickel's worth of weight or pressure at any time to a dog or cat. Even with a horse, you need not apply as much pressure as you might think. You can spend as much time on the ears and base of the ears as you like, particularly with most dogs. These animals are very sensitive and have many of their reflex points in their ears and paws that trigger other parts of the bodies.

Still working from behind if possible, massage the muscles over both sides of the jaw with open hands in gentle circular motions.

Calming the Animal

If the dog or cat is fidgeting as you work on it, you might be able to relax the pet by gently placing one hand in the middle of the spine, facing toward its tail. Do not move your hand; just rest it there in a comforting manner. It helps to project comforting thoughts to calm your pet. Your intent and thought forms are as important as your massage techniques and the energy your hands impart.

Treat Like an Athlete

Dogs, cats, and horses are like athletes. They are active and athletic like few people you have ever met. Consequently, they need to be treated like athletes. When you massage those great muscles in their front legs, put your hands into a "V" spread, or "angel wings." You are going to work your joined hands sort of like hinged scissors to perform cross-fiber friction. In this fashion, you are rubbing across the grain of the muscle or tissue. When you put your hands into a V spread, the thumbs form a V. The thumbs open and cross each other. In "angel wings," you place the dorsal surface of the first phalanges on the tissue, with knuckles of both hands touching. Then rotate your hands 90 degrees to work angel wings on the surface of the pet. Another massage technique for your pet's muscles is for you to move one flat, opened hand up the leg of your pet, with your other hand right behind it to repeat the stroke with the alternate hand. Twist your open hands a little as you run them up the length of the muscles, one hand immediately following the other. This should somewhat resemble a barber pole with swirls around it.

Work the front legs to the top of the animal's body behind its head. Work this muscular area with your thumbs or gently with your knuckles rotating in small circles.

Stroking

Stroke the animal hand over hand, the full length of its body from the back of the head to the tail on one side of its spine and then the other. This is the proper way to pet your dog or cat. It massages the long muscles that run along both sides of its spine.

Hind Legs

Massage the muscles in the hind legs with finger pads in circles and with joined hands in V spread or angel wings to perform cross-fiber friction. You can also use a technique called compression on the belly of a large muscle by pressing the entire palmed surface of your hand squarely on the muscle and pressing the muscle into the underlying structures in a pumping manner. This compression should be light.

The Tail

Work the area at the base of your pet's tail with little circles, moving your finger pads gently.

Massage the animal's tail gently in a chucking technique with both your hands. Grasp the tail with one hand to support it, and then use the other hand to move the tissue forward and back, working your way from one joint to the next.

Chest

Use soft, circular movements of your open hand gently over the chest area of the animal to help increase blood flow and general circulation. Remember, this is the area of the heart chakra. Your hand should be flat and moving in slow, full circles.

Abdomen

Massage the abdomen with one flat hand in little clockwise circles. Perform these little circles very slowly and gently.

Horse Cautions

Horses might seem pretty big and difficult to massage, but they will stand perfectly still during a massage with great patience and appreciation—pretty much the same way a dog will.

As with all pet massages, become one with the animal that you massage. Go slowly and gently with lots of love and patience. Stay in your zone. When you do it right, you perform a little dance with your massage. You move your hands almost in response to your pet and its needs. Your dance enhances your energy. Your dance becomes your art—your healing art.

There are times, however, when you should not massage an animal. Certainly, massage should never take the place of needed veterinary treatment. In case of fever or open wounds, for instance, avoid massage. If a horse has a temperature over 102 degrees F, do not massage. You do not want to increase blood flow with high fevers or open wounds.

Range-of-Motion

Remember the assessment of your pet's posture while standing and walking? You may be able to improve the range of motion in the limbs of your dog or cat, with special attention to the hind legs that might have been cocked or bent slightly forward. Of course, there is only so much that physical therapy can do for the hip disorders that afflict many breeds of dogs in later years. But gently stretching limbs can improve range of motion and overall posture to some degree in many dogs, cats, and even horses.

You will want to put your back to the animal, as you extend its "problem" limb and move it out and around with gentle, even pressure. In the case of a dog or cat, your patient can be on a table or even the floor and should be reclining on its back, if it is willing to assume this position. Horses, of course, will most likely remain standing and might require a spotter for safety's sake. Trust is the key issue here. You cannot do range-of-motion exercises on a pet without an advanced level of comfort on the part of your pet with the physical therapy and with you.

When you lift and extend the problem limb (the short leg, oddly crooked leg, or leg improperly positioned), you should support that limb with one hand at the base of the limb near the trunk of the body. Then use your other hand to extend this limb and move it gently in a slow circle to extend its natural range of motion. Do not jerk or pull hard. Instead, apply even pressure gently. A little help goes a long way. Do not overlook massage treatment to the hip region while you are focused on this problem.

Myofascial Release

Like range-of-motion therapy, myofascial release therapy on your pet might require an advanced level of trust and comfort. This European form of massage concerns itself with the hidden and debilitating problem of tissue bundling in the body. The theory is that body tissue tends to wrap itself like scars around bones, muscles, nerves, tendons, and ligaments with physical trauma. It is apparently a self-defense response to trauma, but it only causes deeper problems.

Typical bundling can be found along the back, causing spinal problems often detectable in posture or sway-back conditions. It is literally like carrying old problems on your back, pulling you down. Typical tissue bundling comes from any kind of trauma, including both physical and emotional trauma. It can come from an accident, stress, or even an old wound or operation that left internal scars.

It is possible to break down these unwanted tissue bundles with your hands by applying gentle pressure in a downward and outward motion. Lay your hand or hands flat upon the back or any other area of the body that might have tissue bundling. It is best to work from the head of your pet and put your hands behind its head, facing the tail. Apply gentle downward and outward pressure toward the tail, without moving your hands. Hold this gentle pressure without moving your hands, simply pushing downward and outward. Do not force things! In a few minutes, the tissue below your hands might give an inch or two, as the bundling breaks down under this applied pressure. Once the tissue gives way, move your hands a little more toward the tail to work another area on the back. As the tissues wrapped around bones, nerves, and ligaments release their grip, your pet might shiver or whimper a little, remembering the trauma that caused the bundling. It might have been an accident, or another horrible incident that had been largely forgotten and locked away. But the body remembers. All at once, your loved one may recall the trauma that led to this tissue bundling. In myofascial release therapy, this remembering phase of recovery is called unwinding. It might startle you at first, so be ready for it. Just comfort your pet and keep it safe. It might want to kick its feet and wiggle around, as it relives the trauma. Allow it to go through this releasing process.

Myofascial release can be applied effectively anywhere on the body that tissue bundling seems to appear. Fix your hand flat on the suspect area and try applying gentle pressure downward and outward to see whether the area is seized or if the tissue gives way freely. You will know the area is okay if your hand slides a little all on its own with no sign of restriction.

Massaging Plants

Gentle caressing of plant leaves and stems has been known to stimulate energetic response from plants. The research of Cleve Backster, as reported in *The Secret Life of Plants*, proves that plants display sentience and emotional responses that can be scientifically measured with various electronic devices. In fact, plants have demonstrated empathy to people and other life forms and react to stimulus from their loved ones, even from miles away. Plants are very sensitive.

But every good gardener knows that already. Some people with so-called green thumbs can touch their plants and watch them grow to healthy proportions with long lives. Other people, with so-called purple thumbs, will tell you that they cannot touch a plant without it withering and dying almost instantly. Researches like Backster have determined the reason for this. Plants are psychic. They can read your mind. They know whether you love them and sincerely wish them well. People with dark thoughts frighten plants and shock them into dying. Your healing intent and pure thought forms are important when touching a plant.

The famous psychic Edger Cayce, who had a good deal to say about health and healing, touched plants to help heal them. He literally put his hands on the plants in order to help rejuvenate them and restore the life energy force within them. His many successes are well documented and catalogued in the extensive library of A.R.E., in Virginia Beach, Virginia, the largest library of its kind in the world.

I have personal experience in applying healing hands to plants and can report that plants are visibly moved at times with the transfer of energy from the human hand to their leaves. They sway in energetic, healthy response. The only reason more people do not notice that plants actually move is that plant movement is generally too slow and methodical to draw attention. Also, people are not that observant. Certainly, most people do not expect to see plants move. If you think about it, however, plants move all the time. They send their roots down and out to great distances to find water and soil nutrients. The roots of some plants, stretched out end to end, would literally reach for miles and miles. Plants also reach out to the sky for healthy light. So plants are moving in many directions to satisfy their needs, despite a lack of eyes and ears. Not bad for a plant!

Because they are so sensitive, massage of plants should be very gentle stroking, such as fingertip caresses that just lightly touch the plant. It is also okay to talk to your plant and send it thought forms of healing love and energy. After all, plants are sensitive and psychic. They will absorb all of the good love and energy you share with them and continue to share a healthy life with you as long as they feel loved.

I have one enormous, happy aloe vera plant that I bought at a KMart store about 15 years ago. I bought it because it looked so sickly and in need of love. It was one of those three-inch potted plants that they put outside the store and advertise three for a dollar. This one looked barely alive. With a lot of love, healing hands, and gentle caresses, my aloe is now absolutely huge and prosperous. I can barely carry her around to find the best light, but do so with each seasonal change. Sometimes I plant her outdoors and carry her inside for the fall on the sun porch. Then I carry her inside the house for winters under the grow lamps. She has given me more than a dozen baby aloes through the years, and some are nearly as huge as her now. Mamma Aloe continues to thrive and reproduce. She is so happy when I send her energy with healing touch or gently massage her, removing dust from her leaves as I do so. I feel that she empathically shares something with me and returns this healing love energy to me. People note that they feel happy and healthy in her presence.

Chapter 6

Helpful Props: Crystals, Water, Music, and Color

You can find many useful props for empathic healing to help your pets and plants. One of the most helpful things to assist you in your energy work will be simply a quiet room with a soft pad or table. Other props might include crystals, water, candles, and healing music. There is nothing strange in any of this. These things are natural to those who are healthy and also companion tools for the natural healer.

It must be emphasized, nonetheless, that natural healing relies basically on an empathic transfer of energy through healing hands or focused thought forms. Everything that is added as a tool or prop simply enhances or amplifies the experience in some way. They have an impact on the presentation, but effective empathic healing can be done without them. This distinction is important, because some people become so involved in the drama of the presentation that they place excessive value on the importance of these props in the delivery technique. A crystal can do little to help you assist your sick friend to heal, unless you program it with your intent and hold it in your healing hand in a focused manner.

Gifts from nature, such as crystals, can assist the empathic healer in the natural healing process. To prepare these tools for the work of natural healing, the empathic healer must go through a little ritual to bless them, consecrate them, and charge them for the shared work ahead. Any shamanic or folk healer from the old world style of natural healing knows these steps and follows them. To do less is to disrespect the forces of nature, and that will not win their support. Since the natural healer seeks to heal with the energy of nature, not having full support from nature could present a definite problem—like trying to start your car with no charge in your battery.

Consecrating Tools of Nature

Whether you are using a healing stone, a candle, incense, or a table, remember respectfully that your tool comes from nature. This is true also for the sacred space and music used for healings. It all comes from nature and the divine universe and deserves to be honored as a noble assistant in your healing work. Do not treat any of your props as things or common tools to do your bidding. Treat them with respect and reverence to honor them and their origins.

Remember at the outset to thank nature and the divine universe for these gifts of spirit. You honor these gifts of nature in this manner. It is okay to speak words aloud to do this or to quietly give thanks. Spirit hears your deepest thoughts when you project them with deliberation. Just say it like you mean it, in a way that feels right to you.

Next, consecrate the prop that you wish to use in your natural healing effort. You can do this by blessing or charging the object for the work that you are about to perform with it. You can charge the object by holding it in your hand, if it is small, or holding it in your mind, if it is large. If you are consecrating a space for your healing work, then you should be in that space when you do so. You can charge an object or place by holding it in your mind's eye with quiet and intense thoughtfulness. Meditate on the object or place. Visualize it being used to assist you in your natural healing work. Project the full force of your will to empower it for this purpose. Focus your intent on sending this charge to your enlisted assistant, whether it is a stone or a chair.

If you do this little ritual properly, you will enlist the power of nature and the basic force of the intent locked in these tools. You will tap into their secret natural powers.

Crystals and Other Healing Stones

Many natural healers are fond of working with clear quartz crystals, and will hold one in their healing hand (normally the right hand) as they work. It is generally believed that the crystal transforms, amplifies, and focuses the energy passed through it by the healer's hand.

Crystals and other kinds of healing stones can be used similarly, of course. The general purpose of holding a healing stone during empathic healing is that the stone's vibrations or energy wave pattern as a potential healing signal or message resonates harmonically with people. But you can also heal with a carrot in your hand—provided that the carrot is properly prepared through consecration and charged with the intent to help you project healing energy. A crystal just works better and more naturally in this way.

Sacred Space

Most people think of sacred spaces as special, often famous sites located here and there around the world. But you can also create a sacred space on the spot for your own intended purpose. Simply give thanks to nature for the site, bless it, consecrate it, and charge it with focused intent and energized thought forms to help you as a power spot for healing. Use your creative visualization to picture the place serving this special purpose most effectively. In this manner you set the stage by programming your setting for success.

Mats and Tables

Bless and consecrate the soft mat or table that you use for healing. If you are going to position your pet or plant on a certain floor pad or table top, then you should treat this setting in the same way that you treat the room or site that you consecrated as sacred healing space. This surface should be intentionally charged to hold your pet or plant in a way that is comforting, calming, and conducive to rejuvenation.

Have you ever sat somewhere that made you feel instantly uneasy? You probably needed to move right away, because the place just did not feel right to you. Well, objects and places absorb negative energy waves from the thoughts of life forms that come into contact with them. They also absorb positive, healthful energy waves from thought forms that touch them. Charge your healing table and healing mats with positive energy and thought forms that enable them to assist you in setting a proper table for healing.

Candles

Candles are great aids in arranging a room for healing. They carry healing vibrations of their own, if properly consecrated and charged for this intent. Select colors that are associated with healing or with the chakras that need attention. Green is an all-around natural healing color for candles. White works well, too, and can substitute for any color (since white is the composite of all other colors of light). Red relates to the lower or root chakra (first chakra). Red in color therapy therefore relates to the reproductive organs, urinary tract, and rectal area, as well as red blood cells. Orange relates to the second chakra and acts upon the thyroid, kidneys, spleen, and colon. Yellow relates to the third chakra and treats the digestive system, liver, stomach, and lymph system. Green relates to the fourth chakra and offers color therapy for the heart, lungs, and thymus. Blue relates to the fifth chakra and acts upon the larynx, thyroid, jaws, tonsils, mouth, and speech faculties. Indigo relates to the sixth chakra and can be used in color therapy for headaches, hormonal imbalances, and developmental disorders. The color violet relates to the seventh or crown chakra and offers therapy for headaches, depression, imbalance, mental deficiency, nerves, and cancer.

Remember to bless and consecrate your candle and charge it with the intent to heal. Then visualize it accomplishing that task. In this way, candles can assist you in your natural healing work with pets and plants or even in personal self-healing. Candles can be burned ceremonially during healing sessions while you are performing other energy work to empathically assist your beloved friend to recover. You could even burn candles between healing hand treatments, although you should be present to monitor the burning candles as a safety precaution.

Healing Music

Healing music works in much the same way as colored candles. Just as color projects light wave energy with certain vibratory characteristics, music can project sound of a certain wave energy. In both cases, the vibratory characteristic of the energy wave resonates with certain parts of the body and can affect healing in reaching harmonic resonance with those areas.

Gentle, soothing music that heals sends all the right notes to all the right areas of the body. The body absorbs this healing energy and responds by rejuvenating itself. It is a bit like hooking up a weak car battery to a battery charger to be recharged.

Perhaps you will use music as a helpful backdrop to your healing session, as you lend your own energized healing hands to your loved ones. Make certain that the music puts your subject into a relaxed and peaceful mood and does not overly stimulate them. Avoid loud, jarring music. I usually play something like Beethoven's Moonlight Sonata, or almost anything by the vocalist Enya. Much in the classical area is suitable, if it is gentle and uplifting.

Water in Healing

The things that sustain life are sometimes very simple. Everybody needs sunlight, fresh air, and pure water. That is true for your pet, just as it is for you. Plants also need quality air and good water. We sometimes forget that in our concern for health and well being. Nature provides the essentials. How could we ever hope to improve on nature?

Franz Anton Mesmer (1734-1815), from whose name we derive the term "mesmerism," was perhaps the first to tap water as a tool in energetic healing. He would fill a tub of water and then magnetize it with his healing hands.

Other researchers in the area of psychic healing have also found magnetized water to be therapeutic. Dr. Andrija Puharich, noted scientific researcher, observed similar success in an experiment with psychic Uri Geller. This carefully documented experiment is particularly amazing in that Geller was able to project a healing frequency from his hands into a glassful of water and have that water maintain its energetic frequency for a considerable time.

I can personally attest to this technique with healing water. A friend of mine in Oregon used to put a quartz crystal into a jar of water and then set the jar out under the rays of the moon. She maintained that the water was being prepared for healing work. She would hold the jar of water in her experienced hands—hands trained in energy healing. The next morning, she would give the specially treated healing water to a sick friend. I have personally tasted her healing water. It was smooth, sweet, and like no other water I have ever tasted. It made me feel a lot better. It sort of tingled all the way down my throat in a joyful kind of way.

Now the beauty of this is that you can start with any kind of water that is clean for consumption. You will energize it to make it pure. Light rays do that. Your hands do that. Simply put the water into a clear glass container. Then project electromagnetic energy into the water with your hands. You can put your hands into the water to do this, as some researchers have done. Or you can simply hold the glass in your hands and visualize projecting healing energy into the water. It does seem more sanitary to avoid putting your fingers into the water, unless your fingers are very clean. Either way, you should charge the water by visualizing healing energy projected it, charging it with your energy and the energy around you. In a real sense, you are blessing and consecrating the water for a specific purpose. You are also energizing the water by projecting energy waves of a specific healing frequency or vibration. To find the right frequency, visualize healing and wellness. Recall with every fiber of your body how you radiate when you are feeling very healthy. In that way, your body can always instinctively "dial in" the right frequency for healing. It is really not so hard to achieve. Every mother instinctively finds it when she kisses a child's wound to make it feel better. Wild animals do this for their young, too. It might sound mysterious and mystical, but it works so well that mothers for centuries have done it instinctively, regardless of their cultural orientation.

Healing water will work for both your plants and your pets. Every body needs pure water. Like waves in the ocean, your healing energy waves will remain in the water for a good long time until they reach their target. Water is an excellent conductor in this regard and will retain the charge or healing signal put into it for many hours, as the water is consumed and absorbed through the body of your pet or plant.

Chapter 7

The Magical Use of Voice

The empathic healer can employ voice as a supplemental aid to healing hands and other forms of energy body work. Your voice, after all, conveys your intention and emotional energy. It also conveys your concern and sets the healing subject at rest with a feeling of calm and assurance. Most importantly, perhaps, voice carries energy in the form of sound waves. With focused intent, you can charge these waves for specific healing tasks. You can direct them at targets you select for healing. You can attune yourself vocally for the intentional, focused activity of healing and send your healing sound waves directly at your loved one.

The use of voice in empathic healing is all of these things, and more. Anyone who has tried to assist a twisting stallion or calm a dying dog knows what voice can add in empathic healing. It can make all the difference.

Soothing Voice

The voice can be soothing and comforting. This is true of a dove's coo or a cat's purr. It is true also of the human voice when focused with this intent. Simply talking to your ailing pet or plant could make it feel safe and secure in your presence. This is important if you are approaching them with healing hands or other forms of energy healing. There is nothing dangerous or particularly threatening about any of the natural healing techniques used by empathic healers. Nonetheless, a sick puppy is a sad puppy and is probably stressed emotionally even before you approach it to help. When you attempt to do something to your sick friend that is unfamiliar, it may become even more uneasy. Physical illness is traumatic. Consequently, your soothing voice may put your ailing pet or plant at ease with your presence and the energetic healing that you are attempting to perform.

Plants like to hear your voice, too, if you are pleasant and soothing. The research of Cleve Backster and others indicates that your plants can become very attached to you emotionally. What you say to your plants impacts their emotional and physical well being. Does that really surprise you? Surely you have noticed how your plants seem to grow better when you are happy, but droop and even begin to die when you are depressed.

As a result of the findings in *The Secret Life of Plants*, many people began talking and even singing to their plants in the 1970s. It became "cool" to bond with your houseplant, which for many people became more than a just pretty thing in their house or a hobby in horticulture. Plants took on an added dimension of life and empathic identity. They became someone to talk to, relate to, and share your life with.

Our pets certainly enjoy their master's loving voice, as well. Nothing is so pleasing to your dogs or cats as the sound of their own name spoken by the one they love. In fact, it is one of the 25 to 50 words that cats and dogs all know. It is the same with a horse, of course. They all know and love their names, even if they did not pick them out. What they really love, of course, is the sound of your voice speaking to them. It matters not that they understand little of what you might be verbalizing, since they communicate non-verbally. Hearing your voice perks up their spirits, which helps them rejuvenate and begin the self-healing process.

Use your voice wisely when speaking to your pet or plant during healing. Use a soft, even tone of voice without any shrill sounds, excitement, or fast talking. Use full, rich sounds instead of crisp, sharp sounds. Speak slowly and establish eye contact without staring. And, yes, it is okay to sing to them to calm them. Our pets and plants love to hear us sing soft, gentle songs—

especially if you can incorporate their names. If any of this sounds odd to you, just put yourself in their place. People who are sick or dying want personal contact and somebody to talk to them in a reassuring way that puts them in a state of peacefulness. This is how we center ourselves as a prelude to focusing our intent to reenergize. All of life is pretty much the same. Just look at your dog or cat sometime. They are pretty much like you, except that they use all four legs to walk, while you attempt to balance on two. We're not all that different.

Tone and Chant

You can use vocal toning and chant for healing. Tibetans and others have done so for years. The harmony of your voice resonates with your body to strengthen and energize it. Resonance unites and holds things together. It is the opposite of disharmony or dissonance that jars and breaks things apart. Buildings can be toppled by the destructive use of disharmony. The loving power of harmonic resonance can be just as powerful in rejuvenating ailing bodies by establishing empathic energy waves of sound that bolster the basic structure of the healthy body. The tone and chant that you employ empathically for your ailing pet or plant should be healthy sounds. Broad, full vowel sounds are good. Rich, deep sounds are helpful, too. Sing these vowel sounds slowly from a place deep inside you. Avoid sharp, shrill, excited sounds. You are singing to the spirit within, communicating on a spirit-to-spirit level. Intone and chant these rich vowel sounds with reverence and meaning. Focus your intent. Project your vowel sounds from deep in your belly to fill your lungs with air from deep inside you.

The breath of life flows in each of us. It can be shared and given as a gift of spirit. Reach deep into your lower abdomen to drive the full force of your energy from your body to that of your ailing friend. It is here that the human force of the will is centered.

Hold your vowels in long, broad tones. Sing the vowel sounds as long as your air and life force will allow you to hold each note. It is best to remove your shoes and sit on the ground. You can assume a perfect lotus position, if you are comfortable doing so. Keep your back stiff and head erect. Focus your attention on the single act of chanting these broad, rich vowel sounds deeply to project the harmonic resonance of your energy sound waves. You should be quiet and meditative during this chanting.

The tones that you project in your chanting will help tone the body of your beloved friend. Empathy for your friend may encourage your spirit to put you into this meditative state to begin healing chants. Spirit, in a real sense, is moved to sing. But spirit always moves with focus, intent, and power. When spirit calls you to sing for your friend, be ready. Do not be embarrassed if you do not have the best voice in the world. It is the very voice that your friend needs at this critical time—perhaps the best voice to do the job.

Harmonic Overtone Chanting

Chanting with harmonic overtones is similar to other forms of toning and chanting. Overtones can be achieved with a little practice. You will need to practice singing simultaneously with your mouth, nose, and throat. Now, everybody sings through their mouth. We are often taught in early singing classes not to sing with a nasal quality. And everybody naturally uses the throat to sing. So what is so unusual about using the throat and nose to sing? Tibetan monks (among others) practice a form of throat singing in which they consciously sing from the throat, as well as from the mouth and the nose. The result is that slightly different sounds come from all three music centers—the mouth, nose, and throat. The combination of these three similar yet different sounds creates a unique harmony of vibrations that is quite powerful in terms of sound energy waves. The overlapping sounds create a harmonic overtone.

What does this sound like? Harmonic overtone chanting tends to sound deep, nasal, vibratory, and powerful. The notes are held a long time, with breath control that opera singers might envy. The great Tibetans who have mastered the technique of harmonic overtone chanting can hold notes in their chants for a very long time, creating powerful vibrations that are obvious to the ear.

These vibrations, of course, are energy sound waves that are designed to create harmonic resonance to help the body heal and rejuvenate. The energy of the healing chants reactivates the natural energy within the body of the ailing subject.

Distant Chanting

While healing chant is usually done in the presence of the ailing subject, often as a supplement to other energy body work, the empathic healer can also help a sick pet or plant heal from a distance. This is especially helpful when the healer cannot reach the subject with healing hands or other body work.

Energy sound waves can travel a great distance. They ride freely on the air. You can enlist the assistance of the winds to carry your energy sound waves by blessing the winds and invoking their kind help. Project the energy as it leaves your body with the force of your will and the focus of your intent. Picture in your imagination exactly where you want the energy to go and the subject that the energy is intended to reach. Visualize your energy reaching and helping this individual. Empower it and drive it from your body with the full force of your will by visualizing the will center in your lower abdomen.

You will probably want to perform your distant healing chant outdoors, standing up, and pointing in the direction where you want the energy sounds waves to travel. Bless the direction that you have selected, and bless the wind that you invoke to assist you. Thank the wind and then request its kind assistance in your focused intent.

As you chant in the direction of the subject you wish to aid, you should visualize that subject and the sound energy being received by that subject in a helpful, healing way. Picture in your mind how your energy harmonically resonates with the subject's body and activates the natural energy forces to begin self-rejuvenation.

In addition to vowel sounds, you might also try chanting the name of the pet or plant that you intend to help. Your plant might not have a name like your cat or horse, but you can visualize this plant in your mind's eye while chanting "violet" or "English ivy." The deva (elemental spirit) of the violet or ivy will help you sort things out in an efficient manner.

In fact, it is a good idea when attempting to help a plant heal in this manner to invoke the deva of the particular species in the same way the founders of famous Findhorn gardens in Scotland did. They communicated with the elemental spirits who oversaw the natural development of the plant species in their charge. As a result, their garden grew to magnificent proportions that astounded the whole outside world. The many forces of nature are at your assistance, if you only ask kindly and with focused intent.

Magical Voice

The voice can be a magical instrument indeed. It can transform and cause change through the creative movement of energy.

Developing your voice as an effective magical tool requires practice. Your voice conveys more than the meaning of words and the accent or pattern of speech that is your individual signature. Your voice conveys a feeling, an impression, a tone. Your voice, on a magical level, relays both your deeper intent and the power of the energy sound waves that are driven by your inner life forces. You must practice speaking in a magical voice with the visualization inside your mind's eye that your voice carries power of energy and intent to bring about specific changes. If the change you desire is healing by energy in your pet or plant, then direct that intent with the full force of your will center in the area of your lower abdomen. Visualize the energy leaving your body in the sounds that you utter, and visualize these energy sound waves reaching the subject that you intend to help heal. Finally, visualize the energy acting positively on your beloved friend, bringing a state of healthy rejuvenation to your dear pet or plant.

Sounds have more importance than the simple meaning of the words that they form. Sounds can have power, if you get out of the way as speaker and surrender the role of magical voice to the spirit within you. Your spirit instinctively knows how to move energy powerfully for positive change by the use of sound in magical voice. You must get out of the way to let spirit do its job in sending healing energy to the spirit of your beloved. To do this, you must surrender your body and your mind to your higher consciousness in a meditative state. You must enter this state of heightened awareness with the conscious intent to project healing sound to help your friend heal. When you reach a state of heightened consciousness, your higher mind is already programmed with your healing intent. You can do this while standing with a little practice, although most people prefer to enter a meditative state while carefully sitting in erect posture with shoes removed and well grounded.

The Breath of Life

There is intrinsic magic in our breath. After all, it is the breath of life. Each one of us was formed by the breath. At birth, the breath of life must be forced from us to begin our normal breathing. A slap on the bottom usually starts us breathing. When we approach death, we cease breathing. Somebody can breathe life back into us, however, to return us to life.

Many religious traditions describe the beginning of life, when divinity breathed the divine spark of life into our bodies. Without the breath of life, we are nothing.

This holds true for all life. Your plants love your breath upon them, as they absorb the rich carbon dioxide we exhale. Plants and people live a perfectly symbiotic life, with plants turning our carbon-dioxide exhalations into rich oxygen that we can breathe. We need plants for our breath of life; and plants need us for their breath of life. Now, isn't that a perfect marriage? We could not live without each other.

We can also share the breath of life with our pets, as I learned. My personal experience involved three little black kittens who were born stone-cold dead one morning. Their young mother gave birth in a cold room under a bed and then left them. When I found them, they were cold and stiff, and not breathing. They appeared to be born dead.

Something inside my head clicked. I believe it was a quick shift in consciousness. Spirit took over for me, as I found myself doing things that I had never considered before. First, I held the three stiff kittens in my hands. I focused my intent on seeing them alive again. Instinctively, I began to blow on them gently. I blew long, warm breaths upon them, like a tiny wind gust. I continued to hold them in my hands, which were beginning to twitch and grow warm with the energy that I was generating in healing hands. I blew gently upon their tiny eyes, noses, and mouths.

At last, one black kitten started to twitch and came to life. Then another. And then the third came to life. I still think that it was a miracle. Certainly it was magic. And surely it was healing energy on a deep, spiritual level.

I called one kitten Zorro, because of its black coat. I called another Bandit. And I called the third kitten Precious. It is amazing that they lived at all. They started life with a gift of spirit. Spirit's gift to them was the breath of life. Their gift in return was the gift of love.

Chapter 8

A Symbiotic Relationship With Pets and Plants

People enjoy a natural symbiotic relationship with both their pets and their houseplants. Both pets and plants give back to us just as much as they receive from us, or more. This is obvious on a very physical level that everyone can see. It is also apparent in more subtle terms with regard to the energy we exchange and the empathic way we support each other in terms of health and therapy. We need each other.

Much of the symbiotic relationship between people and their pets is physically obvious to most of us. People bond with pets. Often they share a deep love that feels like that between immediate family members. In fact, many people refer to their dogs, cats, or horses as their children. After all, your pet is largely dependent on you for many of its needs, including food, shelter, health care, recreation, and emotional security. In turn, you depend on your pet for emotional support, companionship, recreation, and physical security. Your dog will protect you and even deliver your slippers and newspaper with a little encouragement and training. After all, your dog wants to please you. Your cat will keep your basement clean of mice and amuse you with its sensuous cuddling and creative playfulness. Your horse will plod through mud and rain, even though it may be tired, in order to give you a good ride. It is only natural that you lavish attention and affection upon your pet. The bond between you is very strong. What spouse, child, or best friend could entertain you every day, while serving your basic needs and providing unconditional love? Your pet is quick to forgive and forget any cross word or bad mood that might overcome you from time to time. Few marriage partners could match that devotion.

Plants give us plenty for what they get in return, too. They provide us with fresh oxygen for the stale air they inherit from us. They give us their beauty to enjoy wherever we want them to dazzle us—on the sun porch or in the living room. They provide us with beauty, incredible aromas, and fresher air 24 hours a day at our beck and call. Almost everyone seems to love seeing flower plants and pretty green potted plants. We cannot resist drawing near them to smell, and their sweet fragrance makes our day better. Their essence makes us feel alive and happy. They can inspire us to fall in love with nature, the seasons of the year, or the person who gives us that lovely plant.

In fact, we probably receive far more than we give to our houseplants. Still, they are dependent upon us for almost everything in their lives. Once we bring them into our homes, they are dependent upon us to give them sufficient water, sunlight, and air to survive and grow in a healthy way. If the air we provide is polluted, they will die. If we forget to put them in a good window to catch enough light, they will not survive, either. And they must receive their water and plant food as nutritional supplements in order to live. Once we put them in our homes, we have altered their environment and made them dependent upon us to provide what nature provides freely to plants in the wild.

Gardening is the number-one leisure activity for many people. People love plants and love sharing this special bond. Gardening for many people is a planter box or an indoor collection of houseplants, while others till the soil under the sun. People love their plants.

Millions of people also love their pets and share physical bonds. Almost every family in North America, for instance, has a dog, cat, or horse. Many have multiple pets. Their pets share their lives like a lover or confidant. The attachment for many becomes so strong that people treat pets like people and pets treat people like members of their animal family. Your dog will treat you like the alpha dog in its dog pack, while joining your family as a four-legged pseudo-human. Your cat will treat you like a member of its own pride, while joining your family as a sort of furry, little person. Some horses cry the minute they spot their owners every morning, while attached horse owners suffer separation anxiety the moment they leave the barn. Pets are people, too, as one popular saying goes.

It is almost the same level of attachment for many people who take their favorite houseplant with them when they travel or worry about the care their plants will receive when they select plant sitters to visit their homes when they are apart from their beloved plants. My aged mother aloe vera plant goes with me every time I move. In fact, she rides in the front seat beside me in a place of honor where I can keep a paternal eye on her the whole journey.

These are just a few of the obvious connections between pets and their owners and between people and their houseplants. These are physical bonds, for the most part.

Other benefits that people share with their pets and plants in a symbiotic relationship come from the energy we share and the way we care for each other in terms of healing. Once again, pets and plants give as well as they get—often providing more for us than they seem to receive in this friendly exchange.

Energy healing is really an exchange that sends energy both ways between empathic healer and the healing subject. Think of an electronic magnet that pushes and pulls at the same time. That is the way it works with energy healing. The healer shares energy with the subject who is ailing. It might be a pet or a plant that you love dearly. It works the same for all forms of life. Everyone requires energy to live, and the right balance of energy to live well with a healthy life. When an ailing subject that you love receives the healthy energy that you project in energy waves, that subject responds. This is very apparent in Kirlian camera experiments. Kirlian photographs show how a life form receiving electrical stimulation responds by sending back an energy burst itself. It is the same with a person, animal, or plant. Energy and the way it impacts and generates life is universal.

You cannot empathically heal a pet or plant with your energy without receiving healing energy back in return. It is an automatic bounce-back mechanism, telling you that the vibratory signal or energy wave has been received, and has successfully started reactivating the energy within the pet or plant you are assisting. The patient then begins a process of self-healing or rejuvenation. They are self-regenerative transformers of universal energy, dynamos who process energy. But like any electrical transformer or power dynamo, they need a little helping hand now and then, when the energy is not flowing just right. We are the same way. Sometimes we need a helping hand to get energy flowing and reenergize.

It is easy to forget that empathic healing benefits the healer, as well as the subject. We get all caught up in this notion of hero and victim, savior and helpless cripple. Really, we're just exchanging or sharing energy with a friend—a gift of spirit, a gift of love. The energy that we give is never solely ours to keep anyway. Energy is a gift of spirit, available universally for all life to utilize and process. When we give energy in empathic healing, therefore, we do not lose energy. The energy always exists for those who can process it and transform it in their lives.

A sleepy tree on an island in the San Juans forced me to see this simple truth about energy. Some things you can see with your eyes; others can only be seen through awareness—a new way of perception beyond the five senses. Well, this giant tree in the middle of an old-growth forest forced me to see in this way.

I was staying at a wonderfully rustic Theosophical camp on Orcas Island where bunnies run wild and deer walk among the campers in a grove of fruit trees. The camp practices Ahimsa, a Hindu Sanskrit word for "harmlessness" with its reverence and love for the many life forms in nature. I was especially fond of the many old-growth trees in the dense woods that surround the beach camp. I asked a lot of questions about the fauna and the flora at this peaceful retreat. Subsequently, I was directed by the camp's resident manager, Dorothy Abbenhouse, to look for a large, old tree with a special reputation for its wisdom and healing powers. She simply pointed in a general direction at the edge of the encampment, where a small trail led into the dense forest.

I walked to the trail and followed its winding path through the woods. It led uphill, then downhill, and over logs. Everywhere I looked there were large, old trees. The dense forest was already growing dark, and I seemed to be getting nowhere in my quest along this little animal trail.

At last, I decided that I could go no farther without better clues. I stopped dead in my tracks on the trail and pondered what to do next. Then I heard a little voice that touched me deep inside.

"Sometimes you need to get off the path to find the path," it told me. It was so soft and intimate that I wondered whether I had actually heard it right. It was as though my spirit were guiding me, although I had no such information moments earlier. I decided that I should accept this advice on face value. I made an abrupt change in direction, hopping off the little trail and down a ledge that led into a myriad of trees.

I took no more than three or four steps before I bumped squarely into an imposing, old tree. It totally dominated the area. I looked up and knew that I had found the tree I was looking for. More accurately, perhaps, the tree had found me. I am certain that it had directed me there.

I decided to honor this tree, renowned for its healing energy, by giving it some energy myself. I considered this to be a gift to the tree. I put my arms around its massive trunk as far as I could stretch. I projected my love and healing energy into that tree. It seemed to soak it up instantly, as though receiving only a small dose. When I finished, I heard the small, soft voice of the tree speak once again.

“”Now you,” it said. “Let me help you.”

I put my arms around the tree again and felt a huge surge of energy entering my body. It felt warm, tingly, and radiant. It made me feel good all over instantly. I had been tired from the walk, but now felt totally rejuvenated.

I thanked the tree and left, realizing that trees were indeed wise healers. The difficulty for most people, I suppose, is recognizing this fact. They have eyes, but they do not see. They have ears, but they do not hear.

Plants and pets are used effectively in therapy today. Most people will fill a hospital room or recovery room with flowers and plants. These gifts of the garden seem to cheer people up emotionally. Our energy is so tied to our emotions that we even use the term emotional energy to describe how we feel. We feel emotionally energized to look out our window and see trees and flowers outdoors. Many recovery programs put patients outdoors on the grounds to soak up the healing aspects of the gardens. Plants make us feel better. Perhaps this is not surprising in light of the research showing how plants are emotionally connected to people near them and seem measurably upset when we are not well. Plants do care and share their emotional energy.

Pets also have been effectively used in therapy. Dogs and cats are now commonly used for therapy in nursing homes and even in group homes with mentally and physically handicapped people. People pet the cats and dogs and feel instantly better. Staff members in such programs have come to recognize the introduction of dogs and cats as good natural therapy with instant results. Pets are now certified for therapy once it is determined they are easy-going and react well to the heavy physical contact that they will receive.

Pets can empathically comfort us in many ways. I will never forget the way my friend's cat Wizard eased her final days in a hospice bed. Deb had known Wizard for a decade and credited the shaggy, black cat with helping her through eight years fighting cancer. Deb even went on the radio to talk about her amazing recovery. Just when Deb thought her cancer was in complete remission, however, she found herself tripping on stairs and feeling dizzy. It was a terminal brain tumor. Deb spent her last days in a Catholic hospice program, waiting to die.

There can be little comfort in waiting to die when you are only 33 years old. One comfort for Deb, however, was Mr. Wizard. The cat would lie peacefully on her bed or on her lap when Deb sat in her wheelchair. He would not squirm or run around the way cats normally do in strange places. Wizard seemed to know his job. He got close to Deb and just sat there, purring loudly. She would pet him clumsily, and he would purr even louder. At the end of the visit, old Mr. Wizard would jump back into his carrier. The next visit, he'd willingly climb into his carrier at the mere mention of Deb's name. He was Deb's cat, and he loved her. He willingly gave her all of the energy he could summon. Their empathic bonds were very strong.

When Deb died, I had a vision of her walking down stairs in her hospital gown to bring a long, pink ribbon to Wizard's wicker toy box. Later I checked the box. I found a long, pink ribbon, the same fabric that Deb had been sewing into Christmas gifts when she became ill. For weeks and weeks, Wizard would stand at the foot of the stairs at 5:30 P.M. to honor Deb at the time she used to return home from work. He would also sleep in the area of her bedroom where the foot of her bed once rested, long after Deb's furniture was removed from the room, leaving only creases in the carpet. The cat acted as though Deb never left. And sometimes people even heard Deb's TV or stereo coming from the empty room where the cat slept. The empathic bond between pets and owners is very strong, perhaps stronger than death itself.

The Western allopathic medical community recognizes that petting your cat or dog will reduce your stress level and likelihood of suffering a heart attack. Cat owners seem particularly blessed with long life, according to various studies, probably because their cats receive so much gentle petting, which calms both the cat and its owner.

Horses are also recognized for their natural therapeutic value. Horse therapy has been used for many years to help handicapped people. Horses were used early on to give crippled people a sense of mobility. Then they were used in physical therapy programs for mental retardation and crippling diseases. Many people today enjoy the therapeutic help of horses in various treatment programs. Some horses are specially trained for therapy work, although many gentle and loving horses do this sort of work almost instinctively.

In addition to the obvious benefits of therapy from helpful pets and plants, we also should acknowledge the energy that pets and plants give to us. The lift that flowers and plants give the hospital patient could easily be termed a boost of emotional energy. Pets that make us feel better just by touching them could be said to send healing energy our way.

If we can help pets and plants heal by the healing touch and energy that we project to them, isn't it just as likely that they can rejuvenate us in the same manner? Energy runs through their bodies, just as it does through ours. It stands to reason, therefore, that they can empathically heal us with their healing energy, just as we help them.

Empathic healing with energy is a two-way street. When we project energy to help a sick subject to heal by reactivating their self-recovery system, we are stimulating the flow of energy in that healing subject. This is just as true for a collie, mare, or calico cat. I have personally observed in Kirlian camera experiments, replicated by many others in similar tests, that electrical stimulation results automatically in an electrical response. In short, if you stimulate the energy body of a living life form, they will respond by sending back energy. Even skeptics of Kirlian photography call this energetic response to stimulus a radiation discharge. But what is curious on Kirlian film is that the energy burst always looks the same. It looks essentially the same with natural healers who have projected their energy onto Kirlian film. The camera does not lie. The energy response from the subject stimulated by energy looks the same as the energy projected by the empathic healer.

So the empathic healer who projects healing energy to help rejuvenate an ailing friend, whether pet or plant, will receive healing energy back in return. This is like instant payback. It is automatic and free. It is a feedback mechanism that clearly demonstrates how freely energy flows in our world and how lovingly it is given, received, and paid back.

The empathic healer, therefore, will be twice blessed for the act of helping. The first blessing is for the act of kindness, a somewhat intangible gift. The second blessing is more tangible—feedback energy received from the healing subject. As you seek to heal your pets and plants empathically, they will naturally send healing energy back to you. So do not think that empathic healing through energy body work is personally draining. On the contrary, it is energizing for both parties.

Chapter 9

Consciousness, Sentience, and the Souls of Pets and Plants

It has become unfashionable in recent years to believe that animals have souls, sentience, or consciousness. Fortunately, this is not true of all people everywhere, but certainly of many people in the West. We must remember, however, that the Judeo-Christian story of Noah and the great flood shows a God who would preserve representatives of all of the non-human animals on earth, while permitting all humans except Noah to perish. So even traditional Western religion sees non-human animals as most worthy of protection.

Many religions and philosophies recognize the eternal spirit in non-human animals. Native Americans traditionally see the Great Spirit in all animals, trees, and plants. The Celts viewed trees, in particular, as evolved forms of life. In Hinduism and Buddhism, non-human animals are revered as connected life forms, and it is believed that people reincarnate into other animal forms. Similarly, the ancient Egyptians believed that a person who lived an exemplary life might be fortunate to reincarnate into the body of a cat. The European pagan tradition views the heavenly afterlife that people share with their pets as Summerland. There, people unite with their pets in death across a rainbow bridge. Even in Western society today, many case studies of ghosts include substantiated accounts of pets who stay near the people they loved after giving up their mortal coils. Death has no hold on any of us. The energy that flows in human beings also flows through non-human animals and plants. This universal energy defines our uniform spirit bodies.

Dogs often mourn their owners' deaths and have been known to linger at their graves. Cats like my friend Deb's cat, Wizard, continue to observe a ritual in honor of an owner, long after they know that owner has died. Herd animals have mysterious rites to celebrate death as well. Elephants routinely return to elephant burial sites, many miles out of their way, just to stand quietly and reverently over the bones of deceased relatives. When animals behave this way with ritual and mysticism about death, can anyone really believe that non-human animals have no souls or eternal spirits? These animals act as though they do.

I have personally observed this behavior even in salmon. It is common among anglers who fish "for fun" to pretend as though fish have no feeling when they are hooked, dragged into a boat, and then clubbed or left gasping to die. Scientists are beginning to see that fish do have feelings, however. All life forms, of course, have energy, which is experienced on a basic level as emotional energy. All living animals, including fish, have nerves. These nerves relay impulses throughout the body as triggers or signals, including the feeling of pain. Because they do not speak to us, we do not witness their suffering and thus wrongly conclude that they cannot feel pain. But it is really a case where we do not listen. Animals speak in sophisticated ways that most people do not comprehend. They certainly communicate with others in their animal family.

Back when I used to fish and hunt (primitive "sports" that I have since abandoned), I fished the beautiful waters of southeastern Alaska. I'll never forget one summer night there when I fished by the light of a full moon in my open skiff. It was a night that changed my life forever. I hooked a salmon and pulled it to the surface to net. In the moonlight upon the water, I saw that a whole school of salmon had followed this lone salmon to the surface. They watched me as I netted the fish and continued to watch me even after the fish was taken from the water. Their little, questioning eyes stared up from the surface of the water, looking into a waterless world they did not seem to understand. They seemed genuinely concerned where this salmon from their group had gone and what would become of it in the hereafter. In time they could see that there were no answers coming from the surface where I floated in my boat, and they all swam away.

Is this the behavior of life without sentience? Of course not. Sentient life is self-conscious of its place in the scheme of things and wonders basic questions about its existence, purpose, and where it is going. I have never met an animal or plant that did not seem conscious of these basic questions. Have you?

Plants most certainly display sentience, according to the remarkable tests measured by Cleve Backster and other researchers. Plants display concern about others, deep thoughts about death, and empathy for their own kind and even other species. That is almost more human than most human beings you might encounter.

Plants, in fact, display an amazing depth of consciousness. Without eyes, fingers, or limbs to guide them, they reach around corners in dark rooms and alleyways to find light around the uncertain bend. They have an uncanny ability to figure out where the light can be found and will patiently send out runners or bend in the direction of that mysterious light. Could people in a dark room or alleyway find their way through a labyrinth? We would find this difficult, even with decided advantage of our arms, legs, and eyes. Plato pointed out years ago that people are easily confused in the darkness of a cave, where they are apt to mistake shadows on the wall for real beings.

Plants can also find water where there is none, something that people find difficult even with our physical and technological advantages. Plants send out roots in all directions, for amazing distances when necessary to find water. In fact, the composite root systems of some trees with all their intricate fibers would stretch end to end for many miles. They do this with an awareness that goes beyond what people seem to possess. Obviously, they have a special kind of consciousness.

Our pets also display a special kind of consciousness. Their instincts are a special sort of awareness that people might be tempted to call psychic. Many pets are psychic by human standards, of course, as proved in the many accounts in the book *Psychic Pets & Spirit Animals*.

I know this from first-hand experience with my 300-mile cat Mildred. I got Mildred, a tortoise-shell kitten, when I lived on an island in Alaska. She had been rescued, like many lost cats and abandoned litters along the dock streets, by the wife of the regional fish and game biologist. This woman would search for cats that needed homes in a fishing village where big wharf rats played freely under pole buildings and in the rocks when the tide went out. She appeared in front of the little office where I had my newspaper one bright day and asked if I would like to adopt one of the kittens in a cardboard box she carried. I choose the feistiest one, who was bashing all of the other kittens in the box.

Because she took charge of everything and everyone around her, I named her Mildred, after the highest-ranking woman bureaucrat on the island—our local postmaster. In rapid time, Mildred had taken control of my little newspaper office and the chamber of commerce office that was also housed in the building. She loved to wear hats and would leave whatever hat I put on her head all day. Her favorite was the fire chief's hat. She would sit atop the chamber's big rack of tourist brochures for people off the Alaskan island cruise ships, as though she were in total charge of the place. If people moved too quickly in putting a quarter in the honor box on the counter to buy a paper or grabbed a tourist brochure in a way she did not like, Mildred would jump down on the table in front of the rack of brochures and bite them. Once she sent a man who spoke only Norwegian to the hospital, I was told. But that was Mildred.

When I sold the paper and began working across the country, Mildred came with me—probably to keep me under control. Whenever I stayed at a roadside motel, I would just leave the door to my room ajar for Mildred to come and go. She never got scared, and she never got lost. Often I'd find her waiting for me atop the hood of my car in the morning, when I would leave a roadside motel in the middle of nowhere.

When I decided to take a new job at a newspaper in Oregon, I had to pick Mildred up at my parent's farm in northwest Washington State, where she had spent her summer vacation catching mice and grasshoppers in the tall grass. Mildred got upset about something at the first traffic light we encountered in leaving that rural Washington town, however, and somehow slipped out the car through a thin crack in the window. I pleaded with her to come back to the car or let me pick her up. The last I saw of her, however, was her backside. She growled and hissed and me, as she ran back toward my parent's farm house. Well, I figured I could pick her up later. I had to get to the airport in Seattle to meet my son's flight from Alaska and could not wait for Mildred's sour mood to change.

When I called my parent's house later that night, however, they said that Mildred had never returned. They continued to keep a watch for her, but they never saw her again.

Mildred turned up a few weeks later at my brother's apartment in Eugene, Oregon. My brother said that he heard a cat howling at his door one day and opened it to find a tortoise-shelled cat that looked exactly like Mildred.

"Mildred?" he asked.

The cat jumped up and bit him.

I figure that Mildred followed us all the way down Interstate 5 across the border to Oregon, but failed to turn left at Mount Hood to my Oregon home. Instead, she continued due south to Eugene. Why? I had visited my brother in Eugene in the little sports car that Mildred knew all too well.

There are many stories like that about dogs, cats, horses, and other pets who found their way home across staggering distances—even some who found their owners in new locations where they have never been. You probably know somebody yourself who has a similar story. In all of these stories, of course, the pet in question overcomes amazing odds in finding home or owner without a car, a map, or a compass. So how do they do it? We could not do it.

We cannot find our way through a maze ordinarily, either. But the simplest animals seem able to do it. One of my cats was trapped in the rafters of our house when I was a boy, but found its way through the maze when I stood there tapping on a board. It knew that I was there somewhere and somehow negotiated its way through a maze of switchback passages in the rafters to find me. I do not believe I could have done that so easily.

Animal researches such as Beatrice Leidecker and Penelope Smith have documented cases to demonstrate that our pets communicate telepathically by sending and receiving thoughts without verbal speech. That is a lot more sophisticated than the way people utter a series of specific sounds that must be learned as a new language in each new social setting. Animals simply project pure thought forms. No wonder sea mammals like dolphins and orcas score so well on the intelligence tests we give them without any prior socialization. They are operating in a state of higher consciousness that few people ever reach. Whales can even communicate from one ocean to another. Orcas can project a narrow energy beam to kill salmon at a distance with pinpoint precision.

Our pets certainly dream, entering another level of consciousness. If you've ever watched your pet sleeping, surely you've seen its legs kicking at times, as though running. Perhaps it made sounds, as though interacting with others in a dream state. Dogs growl, and cats twitch nervously in their sleep, as though acting out behavior in another realm of consciousness reached during dream state. Doesn't this suggest that our pets are sentient, conscious beings with a sense of spirit existing outside physical reality? When a human's consciousness leaves the body to enter other realities outside the physical realm, we commonly call this soul travel. Since animal consciousness leaves the physical realm in the same manner, it is only reasonable to conclude that non-human animals have souls, too. Maybe it is easier to discuss this common aspect of our being as life essence, spirit body, or life force. Whatever you choose to call it, it is apparent that our pets have it, too. All of life has it. Life force or spirit is universal and common to all life.

Plants have a sentience and consciousness that seems beyond that of people at times, too. I remember a huge plant that belonged to a pair of designers at Home Planners where I worked in Michigan in the mid-1980s. They gave it a little water now and then primarily in the form of cold coffee left in their cups at the end of the day. The plant wrapped all around the large room they shared with drafting tables in its quest for light. The plant might not have started its life in the office with the best lighting, but it eventually wrapped around the entire room to find the large windows on one wall.

When the two designers switched offices with those of us who edited their home plans design books and magazines, they considered moving the plant. Then they concluded that the plant had found its own comfort level there in that room and should not be moved. The plant had a focused intent and projected will to match its intelligent and patient approach for adapting to its environment. That demonstrates an advanced level of self-realization that many people long to reach in their personal evolution in consciousness as sentient beings.

Plants seem much more evolved in terms of consciousness than people in many ways. Navy researcher Eldon Byrd replicated many of Cleve Backster's amazing experiments with plants showing their awareness and empathy with others. He also showed how plants would begin to faint upon perceiving even the intent of a person to injure them. It is obvious, based on clinical research, that plants are sensitive psychics and operate on levels of consciousness that most people do not access. They fear death, pain, and harmful intentions, according to these clinical tests. These are indications of sentient, self-aware life with a full range of consciousness and a sense of soul or life force.

Some birds with the physical ability for speech can not only mimic words, but carry on conversations. Anyone with a parrot knows they can use words that they have learned from people in appropriate situations when they want to do so. I learned the hard way that crows do this, too.

I used to volunteer helping feed birds that had fallen from their nests or broken wings and needed some temporary care. This seems to happen a lot in the spring. Keeping up with their feeding schedule could be quite a chore. A person could walk from cage to cage in a circle around the room, completely losing track of time and place. You just tried to keep pace with the need for these hungry birds to eat. Young birds in particular need to eat frequently and on a tight schedule.

Well, I noticed that the crows at our emergency bird sanctuary were kept in an infant's playpen with a lid to keep them in place. There was also a sign on the playpen, which I did not see. It simply said, "Don't talk to the crows!"

I learned the hard way that crows will steal your words and take over the place, if you give them half a chance. The crows began intercepting our signals and mimicking our speech to cause confusion in the feeding room. I really do believe that they would have taken over the place, if we had let them out of that playpen. No wonder Tlingit-Haida Indian legends talk about the cunning and guile of the raven.

Non-human animals have even learned to communicate fluidly in sign language. One of the most amazing examples is probably Koko, the female lowland Gorilla who learned American Sign Language. Koko is famous for another reason, too. When she was asked by her keepers what she wanted for her birthday at the California Gorilla Foundation, Koko replied that she wanted a cat. Koko loved and cared for her cat, which she personally named All Ball. She commented on the cat's behavior and played with the cat. She cuddled the cat lovingly. One day, however, her cat was killed by a car. The great ape mourned the loss of the cat deeply and would not accept another pet or companion cat for a long time. Koko even reflected on death, when asked to do so in sign language.

All life is sacred and precious.

Chapter 10

Treating Pets and Plants Like People—A Better Kind of People

I can still recall the words of advice that the founder of Pet Rescue in Illinois gave me shortly after she helped me rescue a domestic goose that had been abandoned at a city park. It had been shot by a sick child with a bow and arrow, as it sat on frozen pond, unable to fly away. She told me, that animals were a lot like people, only better. They would suffer in silence, she said, because they are nobler than we are. They would bounce back from abuse and neglect, willing to love and to try again.

That was certainly true of Henrietta Goose. When I found her, she was squatting in a snow bank, where she had collected a huge chunk of snow that froze to her wing, like a block of concrete. Of course, that weight on her wing just aggravated the wound, causing her more pain and making it impossible for the wing to heal on its own. The city park department would not help, other than to offer to dispose of the animal. As in many cities, they assumed no responsibility to feed, shelter, or care for the animals that park visitors loved to visit in the warmer months.

I chased down the injured goose and took her home to my small apartment to defrost her wing in the shower. Then I took her to Pet Rescue, the largest no-kill pet shelter of its kind in the Midwest.

This unique shelter was started as a private labor of love by a beautiful woman who used to appear in magazine ads and television ads as a model to sell Gaines dog burgers. One day, this successful model walked beyond her Chicago high-rise apartment to a nearby park where she found a lost dog. The sad dog was still there the next day, and she snuck it under her coat into her apartment. Later, she found another abandoned animal in the park and took it home, too. Then she found another. Soon the apartment building management discovered that she had transferred animals from the park to her high-rise apartment. So she moved outside town to an old house that was constructed during the Civil War. There, she founded a no-kill pet shelter all on her own. Soon she had approximately 150 dogs, 200 cats, and other exotic animals including geese. The animals spilled over into an adjacent annex building, a trailer house, and sheds. Many of them go to live in foster homes, while many who are not adoptable will live out their lives there.

Henrietta Goose got the royal treatment when I brought her to the shelter. She was rushed to a nearby veterinarian who specialized in putting metal pins in birds' broken wings, often as charity without charge. The goose never made it back to the park or to Pet Rescue. She stayed with the vet where she spent part of her day sitting on a sofa with Tom Turkey watching television.

Because animals are noble and pure in heart and spirit, they deserve to be treated as well as you would treat the best people. For that reason, the volunteer staff at Pet Rescue was told to treat its guests with special care and consideration. The animals were entitled to have a bad day now and then and receive a little slack time on their terms. If one was not responding to the food, we were advised to close down the shelter and take money out of the till to go buy them whatever they wanted in the range of gourmet pet food. "Some days you might feel a little down and need a sundae to cheer you up," we were told. "Well, they're entitled, too."

As similar as we are to our pets and plants, we could learn from them and their selfless love which they give freely without strings. In that sense, they are better than we are. Perhaps we should treat them as potential teachers.

Dogs and cats know approximately 25 human words or phrases on average which they have picked up from being around us, with no formal language training. Horses respond to verbal commands from their owners and have even been known to count by pawing the ground. We, on the other hand, can scarcely distinguish one dog's bark from another. And nobody seems to understand how their houseplant is feeling.

Since we have taken these once-free animals and plants into our homes and lives, perhaps we owe them something more. We can start, perhaps, by giving them the kind of food and nutrition that we expect for ourselves. Forget about feeding them something cheap that satisfies their basic hunger and needs. Think about giving them something good and healthy. Like us, they will be hungry until they get the nutrients their bodies require. Give them nutrient-rich food and quality water regularly in clean bowls, supplemented with pet vitamins daily.

Plants also need more than a little water now and then and also require more than a token spot on a favorite table somewhere that suits your interior décor. Give them plant food regularly, a carefully monitored level of clean water, adequate exposure to natural sunlight, and nutritious soil. Replenish their soil regularly with fresh potting soil and new pots that will accommodate their natural growth. If the sunlight is inadequate, give them a grow light. They give you so much in their beauty, emotional support, and things you cannot even begin to see, such as healing energy and regenerated oxygen. Give them something with love in return.

The same goes for your pet. Your dog or cat needs vegetables, in addition to meat. Of course, these vegetables need to be cooked and ground to a degree. But your feline or canine likes buttered corn on the cob just as much as you do—only cooked and ground to make digestion easier. They also need their greens. They should not be forced to eat grass that has been sprayed with pesticides. They should receive cleaned, prepared green vegetables from you, served with love. You can cook for your dog or cat, and there are plenty of good cookbooks on the market to guide you in the direction of nutritious, healthy meals for your furry companion. How would you like to eat the same meatloaf cold out of a can every meal or dine on the same handful of grains and kibble? Read and ponder the contents of your pet food and consider how fulfilling this sort of limited diet would be for you every meal of your life.

Remember that animals have rights, too. They have a right to be treated with respect and dignity. Do not inflict your values on them too harshly. I knew a former teacher who tried feeding his cat only vegetables, since he was a devout vegetarian. The cat ate the vegetables, including stewed tomatoes, melons, and cooked green beans. But this vegetarian believed that fish was not a meat; and so he would give his cat a bit of tuna and drained water from his can of tuna once a week. The skinny cat quickly devoured this bit of tuna and tuna water, starved for the meat that is needed by all carnivorous felines.

Our pets and plants also deserve a clean place to live. Your favorite houseplant does not want to stay in that same pot of old, stale dirt forever. Repot now and then with fresh potting soil and new room to grow. Your dog might be satisfied with a dirty doghouse or mat in a corner, but don't you honestly believe it would like to have it cleaned occasionally? Cats also need clean litter boxes. And all of our pets need to be properly groomed and cleaned occasionally, though they try very hard every day to maintain their appearance, as best they can. Even houseplants need to be lightly dusted from time to time.

Many pet and plant owners disregard the need for proper shelter and temperature controls. When it gets cold outside, your outdoor plants need to come inside. When it gets very cold, not even dogs and cats with heavy coats are comfortable. Take them indoors in bad weather or build them a properly heated home of their own in the yard. They will persevere and survive only because they are noble, brave, and willing to serve you to their dying day. Make their journey easier wherever you can.

The thoughtful person who remembers to water a plant and put it on a sunny windowsill might forget that their dog or cat also needs fresh air and sunlight. Even kitties in high rise apartments deserve a windowsill with a little sun and fresh air coming their way. Every dog needs to stretch its legs and get a walk, even if it must be on a leash or at a dog park up the road. Let us not make our loyal pet companions into prisoners.

Talk to your pets and plants, and listen to them. They care about you and what you have to say. Do you care about them? If you do, you will share your love and compassion with them. If you listen carefully in a deeply meditative state of heightened awareness, you should be able to hear them. They cry out for our attention, but often we do not know how to listen or do not even try. Their voices can reach a place deep inside us, however, if we get quiet enough to really listen. This is listening without ears, but with your inner spirit and your soul.

As valued members of our families, our pets and plants deserve a calm, supportive home environment that nourishes their emotional needs. Dogs need to bark occasionally to express themselves, and we should make room for these outbursts, which are honest efforts to communicate with us and others. Similarly, cats need their claws in order to be cats. Make provisions for them by clipping back their claws a bit, giving them proper scratching posts, or patiently training them in a loving way to know where it is proper to scratch.

If your dog interferes with your schedule, or your cat's hair clashes with the carpeting, change your life and not your pet. You can brush your cats and vacuum after them. You can work around your schedule to care for your dog or horse properly. It is unfair to force your pet to change to accommodate your every wish and convenience. Remember all they do for us—they guard our homes, catch mice, and provide us with countless hours of entertainment, companionship, and unconditional love.

Some children—and troubled adults—can be cruel to animals without much repercussion. This is a sick way that many troubled people work out their inner frustrations. Until laws protect animals from this sort of abuse, pet owners must take responsibility. And abuse can be more than physical torment, of course. Abuse can be emotional and mental, as well. People should not be permitted to shout at animals or emotionally distress them.

The emotional well-being of your houseplant is just as critical. It is your responsibility in taking a plant from nature into your home and into your life to provide it with a calm and nurturing environment.

As transformers of energy, all living beings are susceptible to emotional crippling. The energy centers in our body transform and transfer energy according to our emotional state. When the energy in our body is low or imbalanced, we become weak and ill. The same is true of dogs, cats, horses, and houseplants. It is true of all living beings. So why do so many treat their pets and plants like pieces of furniture or toys? Spirit dwells in them and works through them, just as it attempts to do in us.

Your pets and plants deserve health and healing as much as any living being. It is important to restore the balance of the natural energy flow in their bodies to keep them well and rejuvenate them when they need it. They will do the same for us, if we establish trust, concern, cooperation, and loving empathy with them. When we care, we share. That is just as true for a kitten as it is for a dog, horse, or a plant that you have taken into your life. They become a part of you.

Chapter 11

Energetic Healing Comes Easier to Pets and Plants Than People

Your pets and plants are naturally better at empathic healing than you are. They live closer to nature and to spirit than you or me. Spirit is that vital fifth element that is so elusive to us, because it is invisible for the most part.

Most people recognize only the four basic elements that they can see: earth, air, fire, and water. Because people are essentially physical beings who cannot see beyond their eyes or hear beyond their ears, they do not know the most important basic element of all—spirit. This divine element magically inhabits all of life, from nature around us to the innermost core of our being. Spirit charges us with energy and allows us to transform with its magic. It is our pure essence, our light body. It is the divine spark of life that makes things come alive. We have it, but cannot recognize it for the most part. Our pets and plants have it, too, and live with it harmoniously.

Our pets and plants heal themselves and everything around them effortlessly. It is a natural and selfless act of love and sharing. That is probably why people find it so difficult. Most people do not act in harmony with nature and do not live selflessly. The fact that you are reading this book shows your concern for other beings, however, and probably puts you safely in the minority. You care for your animals and plants, conscious of the fact that your lives are interconnected and interdependent in many subtle ways. Among these is the energy you impart to each other as natural healers. People could learn a lot from their pets and their plants with respect to natural healing; and beginning to share healing energy with them empathically is a way to learn.

Your pets and plants see you as a part of their immediate family. They are emotionally bonded to you in a symbiotic relationship that has no beginning and has no end. The love flows freely and without measure. This is very different from people, of course, who generally think that they have to pay somebody to receive assistance.

Let me give you an example from my own experience. My old cat, Mr. Wizard, is a natural healer. As I related earlier, he originally belonged to a good friend, Deborah Bennett, who experienced his loving concern during her eight-year struggle with cancer. Since Deb's passing, Mr. Wizard has stayed with me. He was an old cat when I met him 11 years ago, and he is even older now. But he still nurses cats and people wherever he finds them. He seeks out and sits quietly with people and animals who are physically or emotionally ill. His presence alone is comforting. As he sits, his body grows warm, as though radiating energy. He will stay with his "patient" as long as he feels they are ill, patiently working his magic. I have seen him do this with children, kittens, and many others. Old Mr. Wizard is a natural healer with great empathy for energy body work, and he gives himself freely whenever he sees the need to help.

There are many special dogs, horses, and other pets who share our world with unconditional love. The plants who share your home feel an emotional bond with you too. If you have ever put your arm around a tree or put your finger near the leaf of a healthy plant for any period of time, you have felt the energy radiating from these quiet, noble life forms.

Strangely, people always tend to hold back. They approach others with hands closed, not open. When your hands are closed, you cannot lose anything. But you cannot receive anything, either. That is a sad way to go through life, always guarding what little you have in your empty hands. That is not the way animals live. They approach each other and bare themselves. They routinely make gestures to indicate their openness and lack of aggression. We could learn a lot from the animals and plants who share our world.

I remember doing a magazine story once about horses used in therapy for retarded and handicapped children. These were ordinary horses, not select breeds or highly trained animals. They permitted the children to pull on their manes, stumble into them, and just about anything else. The horses patiently waited on the children to mount them, often requiring extra time, patience, and help. Often the horses would lower their necks to meet the children halfway or would crouch down on their legs to make it easier for the children to climb aboard. If the children started to slip off the saddle or otherwise lose their grip, the horses would stop and patiently wait for the child to regain control or get help. These were gentle, compassionate horses with genuine concern for their frail, little riders.

What the children got from the experience was much more than a fun ride. They gained a sense of mobility, a sense of confidence, some badly needed exercise, and a lot of great fresh air on a sunny day. The experience was invigorating for the children, and no doubt therapeutic in many subtle ways. Horses have long been known as spirited animals, and here we see proof-positive that spirit dwells in these noble beasts.

More and more dogs and cats are becoming involved as therapists, too. As true natural healers, they do not seem to require much in the way of training—just a loving heart and patience. Even homeless pets in animal shelters are finding new ways to share their healing love in these visitation programs. Often, a neglected child will experience unconditional love for the first time from one of these visiting pets.

I remember one floppy-eared black mutt we had at the local shelter where I live. Molly was a wonderful dog, but could not get adopted. She had lived in a cage at the shelter for more than half a year, with only occasional 20-minute walks around the block by volunteer walkers. Once every now and then a volunteer groomer would lift her into a tub for a bath and then lower her to the ground to be dried in a small enclosure equipped with a dryer. Otherwise, she existed in a small, metal cage and slept on a cold, cement floor in a lonely part of a building without windows. Nobody wanted Molly. She was no show dog, no pedigree dog, and no particular breed at all.

But she was all love, and showed it when she was given a chance to visit nursing homes. She would nose her way gently up to the old people and rub against them. They would fawn over this loving dog and pet her, and she would let out little moans of joy. Molly loved to visit old, dying people who had so little left to live for. When Molly visited them, the old folks perked up—their eyes brightened, and they smiled joyfully. Color returned to their pale cheeks. The lovable mutt infused them with spirit and improved their outlook. You could just see the energy leaving the dog and entering the people she touched. The energy she shared might have been invisible, but its effect was as apparent and as instantaneous as turning on a light.

I knew a fat cat who became a therapist, too, after her own health came into question. Miss Trixie had lived on the street much of her life, and so learned to gobble anything edible she encountered in trash bags. She never knew when she might find her next meal. When she finally got a regular home, she would only eat at first out of a brown bag tossed in a corner, and drank only out of a vase or flowerpot base. When she finally discovered that food was readily available, offered buffet style to the many animals who shared her new home, she gobbled everything in sight. In time, this calico cat ballooned from 8.5 to 28.5 pounds. Diets did little to reduce her weight, because she had become too fat to exercise—she could only waddle around.

But somebody who worked with troubled children in group homes discovered Miss Trixie one day and saw how gentle and loving this fat cat was. So she tried Miss Trixie as a therapy cat.

Trixie loved the attention and really related to people well. Children could pull her tail, tickle her ears, and even roll her over. Miss Trixie did not mind. She would just purr and ask for more contact. Her presence, it was discovered, calmed the children and taught them how to treat other beings with love and gentleness.

Trixie's owner decided to get her a proper business card. It read: "Miss Trixie, Cat Therapist" on the front, and on the back: "(Please don't feed the therapist.)"

You have probably heard about a female dog who raised a litter of chicks, rabbits or even kittens, often nursing them as her own. We are often told that this is a mother's instinct and not a conscious decision. But animals who are long past the season of motherhood are apt to assist orphaned babies in the same way. I knew one old tomcat who cared for kittens who needed attention, even allowing them to suckle on him somehow. He would clean the kittens, play with them gently, and watch after them.

People have long vilified the undomesticated dog, cat, and horse as vicious and mean, when careful study shows this to be untrue. Such biased reasoning, however, has allowed us to exterminate our natural rivals, since these intelligent mammals have competed with us throughout the years for habitat and food. Well, the wild horse has little grazing land left, the wolf has been virtually exterminated, and the wild cat scrambles and scratches in poor terrain in attempts to avoid conflicts with people. If any wild animals run out of suitable habitat and venture into populated areas nowadays, they are quickly slaughtered.

It is time to recognize that the real encroaching, dangerous animals are people, who have taken from every other animal on earth and given so little back. We should seek to study and imitate the trusting, loving ways of other animals. Perhaps in this way we could learn a natural approach to nurturing and health care.

It is left to our pets to teach us about unconditional love, open trust, sharing, and natural healing. None of them hold back anything or conceal anything from us. They are incapable of clenching a fist in anger or hiding something in their grasp. The peaceful, loving spirit that they receive in their walks close to nature fills them with radiant energy that they share freely. They playfully nuzzle against us, sharing love and body heat. The energy that they process in their bodies radiates from them and fills our lives. In this way, they transform us.

Chapter 12

What We Can Learn From Our Pets and Plants

Much of what we have learned through the many years of human development has come from study of other life forms. From our earliest days as a rather primitive species, humans have been inspired and filled with awe by the majesty of wildlife and natural fauna.

Early people watched the great animals and plant life around them with respect and attempted to imitate them any way they could. Birds inspired us to attempt to fly, and through the years people tried everything from wings strapped onto their arms to finally motorized planes. Similarly, we envied the speed of herd animals like the deer and gazelle and crafted trains and automobiles to move us with similar speed. People have worshipped the craftiness of the fox, the boldness of the raven, the strength of the bear, and the quick action of the cat.

Ancient people saw magic all around them in the forces of the natural world. They worshipped animals as the embodiment of the magic in nature, symbols of this amazing life force. Traditional cultures still show reverence for such creatures as the bear, the raven, the fox, and the deer. To the rest of us, respect for the magic and majesty of nature has slowly died away. We slaughter the animals and trees we could only tame and master through conflict. We no longer compete with any of these incredible animals, despite their powers.

We claim their powers as our own by naming ourselves after them. We name sports teams after them in hopes that they will be as dominant as the eagle, quick as the panther, or nimble-footed as the ram. We put their names on our tee-shirts to claim their power. At night, we dream that we can fly like a bird or spring across mountains like a cougar.

The natural magic of animals continues to fascinate us. People carry bird feathers in hopes that the natural magic they represent will impart power to them. People carry rabbit-foot chains, put horseshoes over doors for luck, and wear animal emblems on their clothing. We proudly drive vehicles with such names as Mustang, Thunderbird, Cougar, Lynx, Sting Ray, Spider, Pinto, Colt, Impala, and Ram. (Curiously, these are mostly older model cars. Less and less do we concern ourselves with the natural world and the power animals that brought it majesty. Now we have cars like Wranglers and Trackers.)

In the movie *Rocky,* an old boxing coach encourages a young fighter to learn to run as fast as a chicken. Try as he could, the ambitious young athlete could not match speed with the chicken, which always outmaneuvered him in training exercises.

Maybe that is the problem. We are always trying to catch the chicken, round up the wild stallions, and cage the tiger. In our wild envy, we try to dominate the animals we admire and cage them, along with the natural magic we wish to possess. Obviously, this does not work. Only by living cooperatively with animals and other forces of the wild can we hope to come into contact with the natural magic of their world. We can only pet the tiger when we have earned its trust and respect. We can put our arms around a tree, climb it, and bask under its glory, only if we agree not to cut or burn it down.

This is what makes a personal relationship with a dog, cat, horse, or even a plant so very special. We can share our world with them. We can live and work cooperatively with them.

I have learned a lot from the animals I have known, and from other animals that have touched my life. They have taught me patience, friendliness, trust, dedication, cooperation, and the ability to forgive. They have taught me when to be quiet, when to speak out, and when to sit by somebody's side in comfortable companionship when nobody wants to speak. They have showed me nobility, courage, and bravery in a variety of challenging situations. Perhaps most importantly, they have taught me some of the greatest lessons in higher spirituality: selflessness, unconditional love, and how to walk in harmony with spirit in nature. Animals have taught me how to live in the moment and become totally awake, alert, and aware.

There is a man who rescues animals in parks and runs a large shelter in California who believes that our pets are angelic messengers who choose to live with people to impart important spiritual lessons. This view is similar to that of a woman who conducts a mail order business in the southwestern United States. She offers reunions with the spirit of deceased pets for closure during grieving. She sees pets as spiritual teachers, since they live closer to the natural world of spirit than people do.

Batman and Robin, Two Curious Cats

My neighbor's noble cat, Batman, was a scrawny gray tomcat who was quite sickly and frail. Nonetheless, Batman protected Robin, the female cat in the household, from neighborhood creatures that frightened her. Robin would hide atop things and remain there as long as she sensed danger. She would not even come out to eat, drink, or use the litter pan. So food, water, and a litter pan would generally be positioned next to her safe perch. Other cats in the neighborhood would find her, sensing her fear and hearing her scream. Just their presence nearby would put troubled Robin into panic. That is when Batman would launch himself to her hiding place to comfort her and show protection.

Batman was a very frail cat who used just about all of his remaining strength to assist his friend. He would lie around most of the day, conserving his dwindling energy, and then come running when he heard Robin cry. Typically, he would fly around corners and leap into the air in an amazing burst of speed and strength. But in the end, noble Batman died a frail cat with a constricted bowel.

All of the neighborhood tomcats, the same ones who troubled Robin, filed past Batman's body when he purred himself to final rest one morning. Each walked past his fallen body and seemed to plant a kiss on the top of his head, as though to show respect. Cats—like elephants—mourn their dead and have rituals to celebrate the transition of spirit. Ultimately, the cats that Batman opposed in defending Robin held no ill will toward him.

Nikki, the Compassionate Dog

Nikki, a female German shepherd and bloodhound mix, was brought into a drug rehabilitation house to provide security. Now, a lot of people will bring home a dog with the vague idea that the animal will bark at intruders and guard the house when people are sleeping or away from home. Well, Nikki sized up the job and decided that she had other duties to perform. She decided that she could help the women at the rehab house on a more personal level.

Nikki did not have a place of her own in that large building with so many private bedrooms. So she generally slept in the hallway or in the common meeting room where her dish was placed. There was a lot of shouting and crying in this house. The women there did not fawn over her, or spend hours grooming and playing with her. These women had personal problems to work out.

Nikki would position herself in front of the bedroom door of the woman she thought she could help that day. She would wait for her to come out, or to return to her room after meetings. Then Nikki would work her wonders. She would nuzzle the woman, encourage her to play, or beg for a walk. There was a lot of love to share. And the woman would walk her in the woods nearby, pouring out love to the dog in return.

It is hard for a dog in such a precarious environment to become too attached to residents who are typically there only for a few weeks. But Nikki eventually came to live with one of the women who went through treatment there.

Nikki was a natural healer. Most dogs are.

Mamma Aloe Vera, a Big Healing Plant

Plants are natural healers, too. My huge aloe vera plant has given birth to many baby aloes, some now nearly as large as she has become nearly twenty years later. I can barely lift Mamma Aloe now. I have transplanted her outdoors in many locations throughout the country, in soils very different from the desert soil she must naturally call home. Everywhere she is planted, things around her grow healthy and strong, it seems. And Mamma Aloe does perfectly fine in Midwest downpours or shady spots in dusty gardens.

I have really tried to care for this amazing plant. But I have occasionally knocked off a part of her when attempted to move her through doorways that are much too narrow for her huge girth. Whatever befalls her, however, Mamma Aloe seems to thrive. She continues to grow, pop out babies, and blossom with a beautiful white flower on a stem each year.

Whenever another houseplant is doing poorly, I place it next to Mamma Aloe. The plant seems to perk up, even if it is not one of her babies. Research indicates that plants naturally relate to physical, mental, and psychological stress suffered by one of their own with whom they relate. But Mamma Aloe seems to relate empathically with many plants that come into contact with her, even new plants that are strange to her. Mamma Aloe must send healing energy to them, as they all perk up enthusiastically and began to look healthier almost immediately.

Of course, any huge and old plant as amazing as Mamma Aloe attracts many human admirers who want to receive her magic healing help, too. Aloe vera plants have long been regarded as healing plants, and for good reason. Just last summer I nearly sliced my left thumb off my hand while attempting to clean a sharp, metal roof at a Theosophical summer camp grounds. I felt foolish, especially when I could not stop the bleeding. I refused stitches, although a nurse on site told me that I needed them. The next morning John Abbenhouse, the former Indralaya camp manager, brought me some aloe vera to put on my cut. Well, the healing was remarkably quick and clean. Mamma Aloe would have been proud.

So it does not surprise me that many people consider my plant to have magical healing powers. Some do not even ask for a cutting to sprinkle the amazing aloe vera plant juice on their wounds. They just sit or stand next to Mamma and absorb her healing energy. They feel energized almost immediately and find the communion to be therapeutic. Many return for more.

We could learn a lot from our houseplants and pets. They are natural healers and give of themselves freely and without reservation.

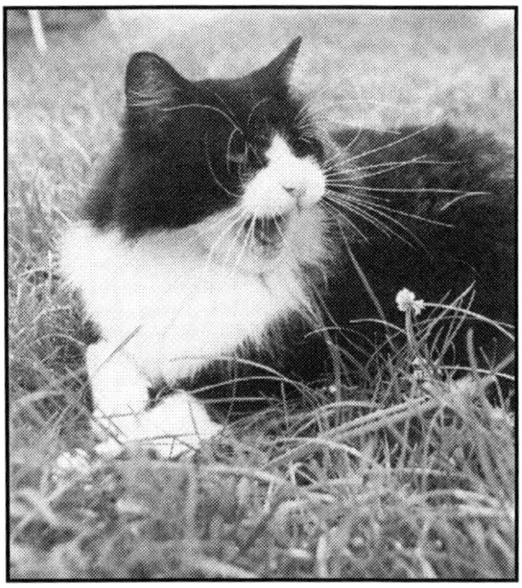

Mr. K, the author's top cat

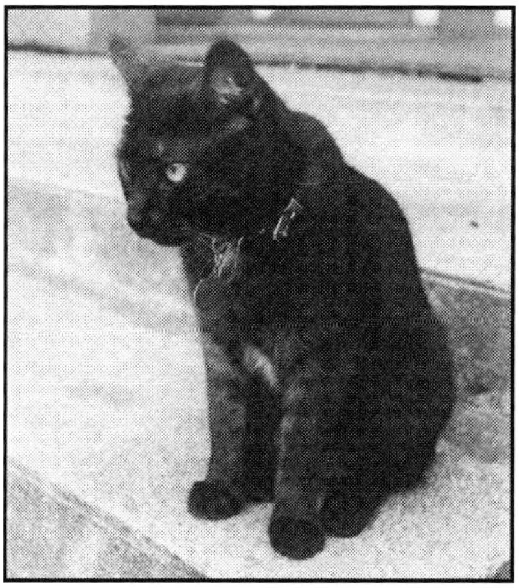

Little Miss Ben, an
amazing recovery story

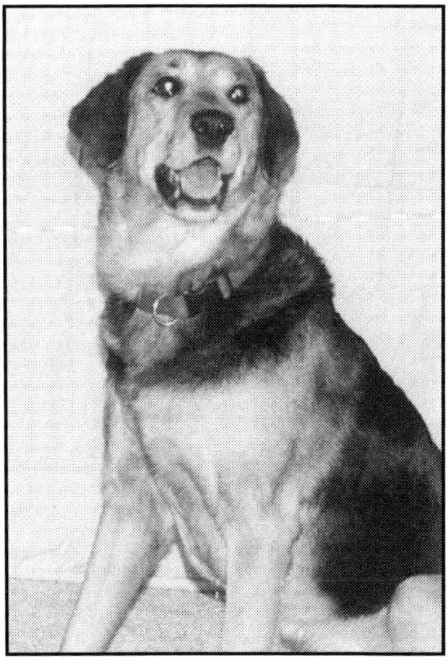

NIkki, the therapy dog from
the drug rehabilitation house.

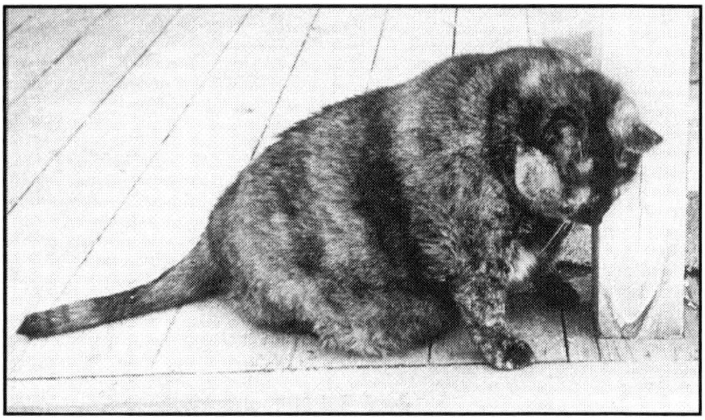

Miss Trixie, the therapy cat

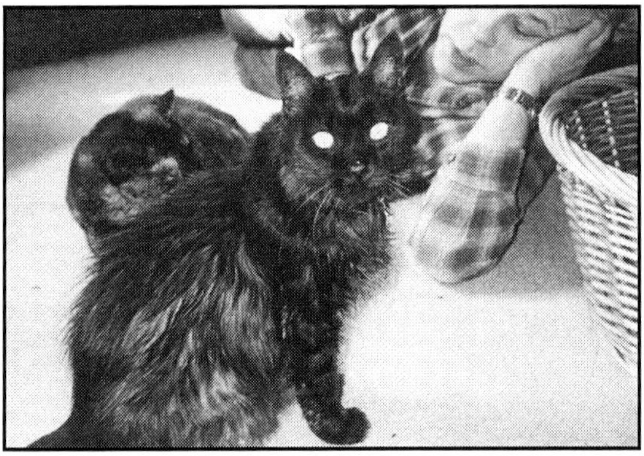

The author with Mr. Wizard, age 20

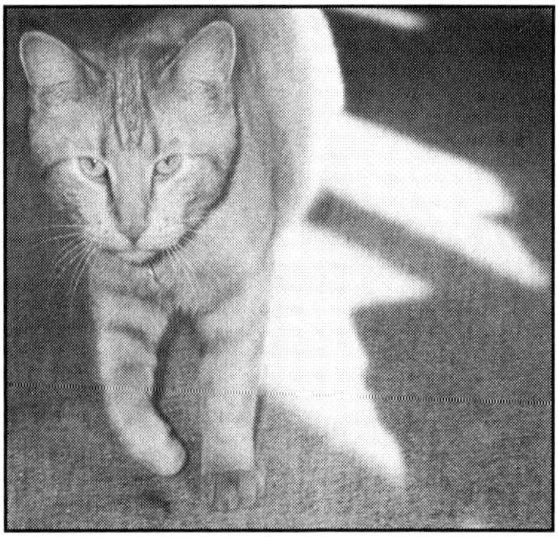

Sunshine Kitty, the author's cat
recovered from the street

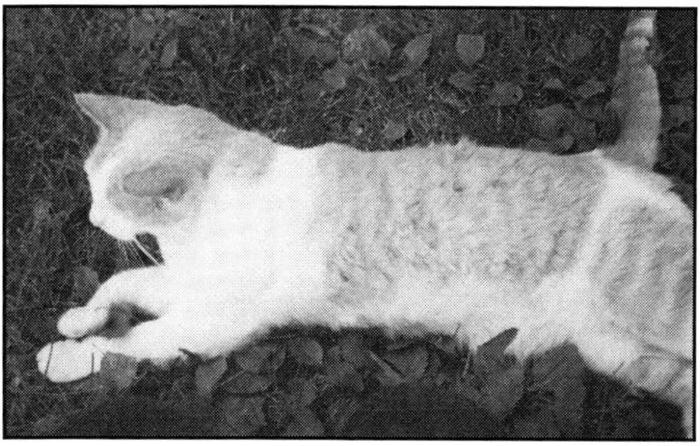

Mr. Peaches, rescued from the streets

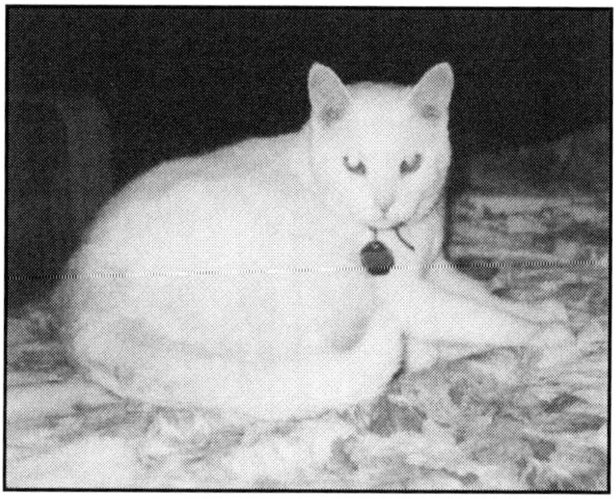

Miss Polly, who showed up on the author's porch one day and stayed 20 years

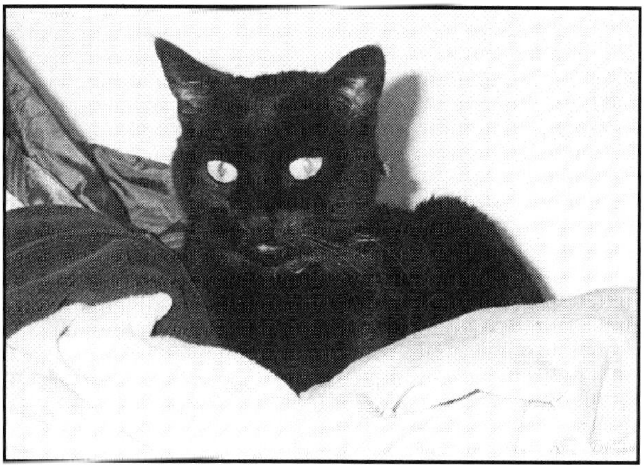

Salvador Dali, born in an old attic.

Chapter 13

Together, in Harmony, We Sing Our World Into Being

You, your pets, and your plants all play a contributing part in a grand universal symphony of creative sound energy. The blending of harmonic voices has always played a key part in our world from its creation.

In the beginning our world was sung into being, according to oral history passed down through the generations by Native Americans and other peoples. This legend makes sense, if you consider sound waves to be invisible energy and harmony to be a cooperative approach that builds bridges. Harmonic resonance is a constructive force that establishes and maintains structural integrity.

Knowing that harmonic resonance creates our world and holds it together is an important discovery for each of us to make—the kind of discovery you make deep inside yourself. It is the discovery that you are more than a lone individual floating through life on your own. It is the spiritual awareness that you are really part of a great choir that has the ability to make glorious music. The music that formed our world as a divine expression can be heard today by those who have the ability. It is an ageless song, a song without beginning or end.

Together we sing our world into being as co-creators of our reality. We do this harmoniously and with resonant integrity, each voice in support. The energy of our thought forms contributes to a great symphony of sound waves. Many voices join cooperatively.

Animals and plants blend their voices with ours. These voices sound silent to the untrained ear. But if you learn to listen to the sublimely beautiful music of the universe, you will hear them very distinctly. You must listen not with your ears, but with your higher awareness.

All living things that process energy have the ability to send thought forms as energy. This energy can take many forms. It can radiate with the properties of certain colors—healing, projecting, transferring, and reaching a designated goal. When energy from a number of sounds has a common goal, purpose, and frequency, then it assumes a beautiful harmony—a resonant harmony.

To achieve harmonic resonance, everything and everyone who contributes to the great symphony must be united in total accord in a perfect blend. The power and magic of harmonic resonance is that the sum of the individual components is greater than the individual pieces. There is added strength in the union and blending of voices.

This is obvious in a choir. It is obvious in an orchestra. Sometimes subtle energy waves are less obvious and harder to hear, however. Few can hear this sort of sound. The mystic can hear it. The spirit walker can hear it. The person who learns to meditate and reach a state of heightened consciousness can hear it. You hear this sound not with your physical senses, but with a keener form of perception—heightened awareness. You must be perfectly quiet, still, and attentive to hear it. You will find it when you learn to reach the still point deep inside you.

The divine music of the universe can be tapped for healing. The natural healer who works empathically with radiant energy learns to feed the harmonic resonance, access it, and tap it for healing power.

Harmony is the soothing voice that comforts and heals. Harmony is the chorus of birds singing together to brighten the day. A world without harmony is a world filled with dissonant noise, friction, and destruction.

The universal music is the most beautiful sound in the world, even though it is hard to hear. Almost everyone has heard it a little at some time or other. You might hear it just when you are waking in the morning, still more in the world of spirit than in the physical world. Or you might hear it watching a sunrise at a time when you are still and very quiet inside yourself. That is when most people really listen and when most people really hear.

Now is the time to listen and the time to sing. Now is the time for harmony in your life. You can contribute to the harmonic resonance of this divine music by remembering what it feels like to be well. That is the frequency that you must project. It is the feeling of a mother who kisses a child's bruise to make it feel better. It is the feeling of healthy daffodils blowing in the spring wind. It is the resonant energy of the planet healing itself after a disaster that levels trees and flattens mountains. This is the energy frequency that you must project to blend with the harmonic resonance.

Your healing thought forms join the universal chorus. They blend with the call of the birds and the gentle love of the trees. Your intentions join with theirs to make music that heals and binds.

Spirit speaks to us in this way. This is divine communication in the universal language of creation—healing music. When we learn to listen to the music of life, we are listening to divinity. At these moments, we are perfectly attuned.

We can sing to the stars, the mountains, the rivers, and the clouds. We can sing to the four elements and the winds. It does not matter, if your voice is not clear and polished. What matters is your intent.

As healers, we can tap the music of the divine by putting ourselves into a meditative state and asking for healing power to enter our lives and the lives of our friends and loved ones.

Animals and plants, who speak without words, find it easier than people to add their energy to the universal pool and easier to draw from its power when they need it. They live in natural harmony with nature and spirit, unlike most people.

Fortunately, people are beginning to learn. And we start with what we know—the obvious, physical world of sound. Many hospitals and therapists today incorporate music in the healing process. Patients in recovery rooms listen to soothing music that helps them heal faster. Soothing music balances the body harmonically. Soothing music binds the resonant integrity of the body, as it strengthens the spirit. Such music encourages patients to recover faster. Music can inspire us, move us, and strengthen us. This is because we are more than physical beings. We are as multi-layered as an onion, with a vast webbing of subtle spirit bodies that encase us. When one of our subtle bodies is damaged energetically, our physical body displays the symptom. Repairing our physical body, however, does not always fix our subtle problems.

It is the same with a dog, cat, horse, or houseplant. They, too, are multi-layered beings with subtle spirit bodies that can become energetically imbalanced or weakened. Illness on the physical level occurs first on another level of our multi-layered beings.

Music stimulates the different energy chakras throughout the body. If we were to hum one note over and over, we would quickly discover the correspondences between certain notes and certain chakras. The seven notes in the diatonic scale correspond to the seven basic chakras in the body and the seven colors of light refracted by a prism. It is just possible that nature is trying to tell us something here. The note "C," for instance, corresponds to the color red and also the root chakra in the body. Rock music generally stimulates the lower chakras, whereas soothing music generally stimulates the higher chakras. Beautiful, pastoral music stimulates the crown chakra at the top of the head.

Musical notes also help to tone the body. This is like tuning a car engine. We can tone the body of a living creature by chanting and holding long vowel sounds. You can feel the deep vibrations of these sounds as they work deep inside the body. Body toning is a natural way to improve wellness and wholeness by restoring energy balance within the body. Think of the chant as a tuning fork. As the body hears the chant, it resonates with the chant to restore perfect pitch.

In harmonic overtone chanting, long vowels are sung and held. With practice you can chant through your throat and nose simultaneously to get rich, deep vibrations that shake the entire body and reverberate off walls and throughout anyone within range. The sounds especially resonate inside the person who is chanting, as that person becomes both the sender and receiver of the healing message. The sound makes you whole and restores balance and vitality to your body. It acts upon all your chakras, fine-tuning them into perfectly orbiting vortexes of psychic and spiritual energy. The very sound of the chanting can put you into a state of higher consciousness.

As discussed previously, you can also chant to send healing energy as a message to another person, pet, or plant.

You can also sing to birds, squirrels, and wolves. Because they walk in nature and live close to spirit, they will hear you. They are already attuned. You can use intonation to convey your message, a conscious intention to heal with sound energy and thought energy. This is the language of pure love.

The classical masters of music seemed to know how to reach a level of divine sound far beyond our physical plane, according to the noted author Helene Corrine. She suggests that many of the great composers seemed to visit the fourth dimension—outside the physical world—in a state of higher consciousness. This sublime music seems to be the most healing for pets and plants, and people as well. Aura readers have noted amazing changes to auras when great classical music is played. To reach the divine source of this inspiring music most people tap into their higher consciousness and leave their body through meditation. Once disconnected from the physical world and physical sensations, the higher mind explores the universal consciousness. Here is where the divine universal music can be found by those who are quiet and patient enough to really listen with awareness. This beautiful music resonates with harmony that binds, builds, and heals. The healer who taps into this music is filled with resonant harmony and can relay that resonant harmony to those loved ones he seeks to heal.

Chapter 14
Practical Applications and Exercises

It is now time for some practical considerations about energy healing. This is essentially a book about energy body work that you can apply to stimulate health in your pets, plants, and even yourself. It should be stressed, however, that your potential application of these empathic healing techniques are virtually unlimited. They can be applied to birds, ferrets, snakes, gerbils, and trees—to name only a few. They can be applied to any living being.

While this sort of healing is natural and has been common in many parts of the world since the beginning of time, it is also inherently magical. It is not an illusion that involves a sleight-of-hand trick. Rather, it is magical in the traditional, serious sense. This is because it involves the creative movement of energy and transformation. Energy healing in its many forms requires the creative movement of energy to accomplish transformation. Hence, it is magical—or magickal, as some have called it. This is natural magic, since it involves the forces and elements of nature. Natural magic dwells in us and all around us. We can access it and exercise it as agents for change, if we know how. It is really not that hard.

The natural approach to empathic healing using energy has several key elements, including heightened consciousness, thought projection, creative visualization, magical intent, force of will, and psychic sensitivity.

Heightened Consciousness:

It is very hard to practice empathic healing and project healing energy from the body to a loved one without entering a state of higher consciousness through meditation. For many people, this sounds almost impossible, but it is easier than it seems. You simply clear your mind and tune out all distractions to reach a quiet, still point deep inside you. When you have cleared your mind, a higher mind becomes super alert and takes over with a new kind of perception. Your body might be numbed, but your higher mind is keenly awake and alert. It allows you to see, hear, feel, and extend in ways that previously seemed impossible. That is because you are no longer limited by the restrictions of the physical world. You are now elevated to the world of spirit.

Exercise—Higher Consciousness

There are many tips on how to mediate. The following exercise is meant to simplify things for you.

Needed:

1. A quiet room with a straight-back chair.(Or a squatting perfect lotus position).
2. Shoes removed and feet firmly grounded on the floor
3. You might want to turn off the lights and close your eyes to make things a little easier, although these steps are not absolutely necessary. (You can meditate anywhere and anytime once you learn how.)

Directions:

1. Sit still and quietly, firmly grounded on the floor.
2. Tune out all external distractions, including your sensory perceptions.
3. Tune out all internal chatter and thought, reaching a still, quiet place deep inside.
4. Focus on only one thought and carry that gently with you in the back of your mind like a picture image of what you want to do. In this case, it will be empathic healing. For this exercise, you might want to hold a picture of the loved one you intend to heal empathically and visualize how you will go about it. Perhaps you will picture doing this with healing hands, or another form of energy healing that is familiar to you.
5. When your mind is completely blank, wait quietly and patiently for a blank slate to appear in your mind's eye. Perhaps you will see this as a void.
6. Continue to meditate patiently and silently until your higher mind takes charge, carrying your consciousness to new heights of awareness.

(Note: If you are meditating as a prelude to performing empathic healing, then you should rise and begin your healing work when your higher consciousness takes charge. You will know this feeling intuitively. You might feel a little disoriented at first, but certainly more capable.)

Energy Transformation:

We all transform energy, which we receive naturally from forces around us. In this sense, we are self-regenerative dynamos of energy. From time to time, however, the energy centers within our bodies become troubled and faulty with energy blockages, energy leaks, and energy imbalances. When this happens, we need an emergency energy infusion. We can accomplish this by sitting in the sun, drinking quality water with plenty of electrolytes, and breathing quality air. Colors revitalize our energy, as do sounds. We can also quickly stimulate the natural energy flow within the ailing body by a personal transfer of energy from another body. Remember, energy travels in many forms. It can travel as sound waves. It can travel through the air. It can travel at the speed of light as healing thought forms encoded with energy. Such energy is invisible to the naked eye. It is a vibration, a frequency, a wave that moves from one place or person to another.

Exercise—Healing Touch:

Practice using your hands to heal with this simple exercise. It will convince you that you can control the flow of energy from your hands to stimulate a loved one in a way that will rejuvenate their energy balance for good health. You can use this technique for your pets or plants, just as easily as you can use it on another person or on an ailing part of your own body. To help you gain a feel for the sort of natural tingling or warm sensation that your hands will feel as bounce back response from your healing subject, practice on a pet or even a plant. To get verbal feedback from the subject of the healing and determine how they feel, it would be best to practice this exercise with another person.

Needed:

1. Another person to assist you.
2. Shoes removed, with your feet firmly grounded on the floor.
3. A quiet room with two straight-back chairs is ideal, but not necessary.

Directions:

1. Face your assistant, with both of you seated in your chairs with shoeless feet firmly ground on the floor.
2. Put yourself in a meditative state by tuning out all external and internal distractions, shutting down sensory overload, and ceasing all thought.

Clear your mind and find a still, quiet place deep inside you. It may help to begin conscious breathing through your nose with deep, slow breaths.

3. Extend your hands to each other, as though to touch them. Do not actually touch hands, but instead keep them approximately two inches apart, holding them in this position.

4. Keep doing this until you both become aware of the electromagnetic charge of energy passing through your hands to the other person. You might feel this as a warm or tingling sensation in your hands. This is the bounce-back sensation, as you stimulate the energy system in your partner. Your partner should feel it, too. Exchange comments on the sensation.

5. Try with your right hand to send energy to your partner's left hand. Exchange positions, with your partner sending energy from the right hand to your left hand. Exchange comments about the different sensations.

6. Follow this by standing behind your seated friend and slowly lowering the palm of your right hand to the head of your partner. Instruct your partner to inform you when the sensation of your body energy is felt on the head, before you lower your hand far enough to make actual tactile contact with the head.

(Note: This is also a good start to a session of healing hands.)

Optional:

If you are without a partner, then try this exercise alone by slowly bringing the open palms of your hands closer together, until you first sense the energy passing from one to the other. (Your hands are a perfect double helix, and ideal for projecting energy to another part of your body, should you ever sprain an ankle or cut a knee, for instance.)

Creative Visualization

Creative visualization is more than imagination, although that is a part of it. In creative visualization, a person visualizes something and then creates that situation. Consequently, this is transformation that involves the movement of energy in a magical way. Everybody can do this. Many people will picture in their mind's eye having a certain person call them. When you visualize it happening and make it happen, you have practiced creative visualization of a very common type.

To do this effectively on command under challenging situations, however, you will want to enter a state of higher consciousness through meditation. Great things are possible in this heightened state of awareness.

You can visualize somebody who is sick becoming well. Picture this loved one surrounded by healing colored light, healing sound vibrations, and electromagnetic energy that you send their way. You picture them needing the healing energy, receiving the healing energy, and responding to the healing energy. This energy is yours to give, but remember that you gathered it from nature around you. Energy is everywhere and can be directed to accomplish wonderful things. We are transformers of energy.

Thought Forms

Thought forms are what you send as focused energy bundles in concentrated exercises of creative visualization. When you intend to materialize something through creative visualization, you need to drive your thought forms to turn them into thought power. Your thoughts then become energy signals or messages that are directed at a specific goal or target. This is a magical display of moving energy for transformation—the kind of magic that anyone can do with proper focus and intent. Natural healers who heal with energy on an empathic level do this all the time.

Magical Intent

To drive your thought forms and empower your creative visualization, you need focused intent. The intent that you carry with you in a state of heightened consciousness is different from the sort of everyday intent that you carry in the normal, physical world of ordinary consciousness. This sort of intent is super-charged and can move mountains. Because it can move energy and bring about transformation, it is magical by definition. Having this sort of magical intent does not make you a superman, wonder woman, or even a magus. Every living being has the potential to exercise this sort of magical intent.

Intent is a combination of focus and will. In entering a state of heightened consciousness to accomplish something specific, you must carry with you into higher consciousness the special *intent* to accomplish that transformation. This can be tricky, because in meditation we seek to turn off all thoughts. The intention of healing must be focused. Carry that one intent with you into higher consciousness as a picture that you do not process or ponder, but gingerly carry as a blueprint image.

Once you enter higher consciousness with this special focus, you need a way to drive this intent to its targeted goal. That is an exercise of will. This is not the same will we experience in ordinary reality, but a magical exercise that moves energy for transformation. Your natural will center is located in the lower abdomen. Do not think of this as your physical body, but as one of the subtle energy bodies that envelops your physical self. You drive your focused intent with will that you draw from that area of the body. With practice, this becomes a natural act whenever you want to send energized thought forms with focused intent. At first, you may feel a surge in the area of your lower abdomen, as your will is projected. This is completely natural. This is a standard part of projecting your energy and focusing your intent toward a specific subject. Your intent will always reach its mark with complete accuracy, regardless of distance or the unknown whereabouts of your subject, since your creative visualization acts as a perfect locator beacon.

Exercise—Projecting Thought Forms With Intent

Needed:

1. Quiet room.
2. Shoes removed for grounding.

Directions:

Enter a meditative state by clearing your mind of internal and external distractions and finding a still, quiet place deep inside you. As your physical body grows numb and your ordinary consciousness gives way to the higher mind, gently carry with you one intent. This will be your focus when you enter the non-physical world of heightened awareness.

For the sake of this exercise, carry a picture of the loved one that you intend to heal from a distance. Perhaps this is a pet. Perhaps it is one of your houseplants. You can send healing energy to this loved one, despite the distance.

When you enter higher consciousness with this intent, your awareness will know what to do with it. This is one of the amazing things about natural healing. In a state of heightened consciousness, your awareness takes charge to accomplish your intent.

The picture of the loved one you want to heal will be crystal clear in your mind's eye, even though you are no longer seeing with your physical eyes. You sense that you can visualize this loved one receiving and responding to your help. It is just a matter of projecting energy toward your subject.

Your creative visualization will find the target for you with pinpoint accuracy. All that is left for you to do is project the power of your will from the lower abdomen area of your subtle body to drive the energy from your body to that of your subject. You are conscious of this force driving your energy and the perfect focus of your intent. You visualize your subject receiving your energy and responding to it as a part of the natural healing process.

Psychic Sensitivity:

Everybody has psychic sensitivity, of course. Some people call it extrasensory perception or ESP. Some call it intuition. Some call it second sight. If you allow yourself to feel things with intuition, you will notice that you are not using the normal perception of your five physical senses, but sensing things on a deep level with a sort of subtle, second layer of perception. This is awareness. It is the kind of perception that other animals utilize to sense a coming storm or disaster around the corner. It is the kind of perception that plants use to find sunlight and water that are outside their immediate environment, as they grow their way around obstructions and stretch their limbs to find what they intuitively know is just around the corner.

Humans probably used our natural awareness on a regular basis too, before we invented binoculars to improve our limited physical sight and fashioned listening devices to improve our limited physical hearing. Now we only seem to see and hear what our physical senses allow us to perceive. If we do not hear something, we just assume that it made no sound. But still, animals hear things that we do not and plants see around corners in ways that we are unable or unwilling to consider.

In a state of heightened consciousness, a person can leave the limitations of the five physical senses behind and tap a greater kind of perception. If animals and plants teach us nothing else, they can teach us this one wonderful way to see the world. Animals communicate without words. Flowers know just when to tuck away safely for the coming of night. They are more aware of their total surroundings and the subtle energies around them. We can learn to do this, too.

The natural healer learns to meditate, visualize, and transfer energy with focused intent through psychic sensitivity. As an empathic healer, you must be sensitive to psychic energy to do these things and empathically share energy. There is nothing mysterious about any of this, once you learn the steps. It is just a matter of focusing your energy and sharing it. Obviously, you must become sensitive to the psychic energy that you seek to share, and sensitive to the loved ones that you seek to help with this healing energy. So psychic sensitivity is really little more than feeling something deep inside you and being willing to share what you find there. It is compassion and caring.

Chapter 15

Some Precautions

You can be a positive agent for change in your world. Keep in mind, however, that there are logical limitations, especially when you are trying to influence another living being to change. At best, we can change ourselves and only offer assistance to stimulate others to change on their own. In the case of empathic healing, for instance, it is important to remember that the sick ultimately heal themselves. Like us, they are self-regenerative dynamos who transform energy as healthy beings. We can aid them by stimulating the natural flow of energy in them, but they ultimately heal on their own. Healing is a process of becoming. This is just as true for cats, dogs, horses, and plants as for people.

There are a number of common-sense restrictions that should be observed by the empathic healer regarding application, technique, and attitude.

The Proper Attitude

First, allow your dog to be a dog and your cat to be a cat. Do not dress your horse like a clown. Do not treat a houseplant like one of your children and carry it around on your lap everywhere you go. If you do not allow your pets and plants to be themselves, you are guilty of anthropomorphism, a sin of arrogant pride in which you falsely attribute human characteristics to animals and other non-human beings.

Certainly, this book has argued that people should treat their pets and plants like people to a degree. But please do not cross this line. Dogs need to bark to express themselves. They like to hang their head out windows, to wander around the backyard sniffing everything in sight. That is being a dog. Do not try to change them by dressing them up, carrying them on your lap in the car, putting them on the phone, or treating them like children. The same goes for cat owners, horse owners, and plant owners. Really, we do not own them at all. We have made a sacred contract to share our lives and homes with them, showing them proper respect and consideration. So respect them for who they are and let them live a normal life.

Remember that healing does not always happen just the way we want. Nature knows better. Your patient often knows better. You will be disappointed from time to time in your work. Sometimes illness is a subtle signal to the sick to take a close look at something wrong deep within them. In such case, the illness is only an outward symptom of a deep-rooted problem. Other times, illness can not be thwarted and will take its toll. It can be the destiny or karma of the sick, which empathic healers cannot change. And sometimes illness is too advanced to alter, regardless of our best intentions. Remember that dying is also a part of living; it is part of the wheel of life. Every physical body dies in time. But that is not to say that the spirit dies with the body, and even the body is "reborn" when it offers the nourishment of its decay to foster new life. Do not mourn your dead loved ones. Death is transition. For those who are painfully ill and tired beyond natural regeneration, death is the ultimate cure for their suffering—a release and an escape to a better place.

Sometimes we try to do too much and put undue burdens on ourselves to make everything right. We cannot shoulder the full weight of the world, but the sensitive healer feels the pain and tries to help. This is both the blessing and the plight of the healer. We must remember that we are only helpers. We can assist and aid, but we cannot change everything in the world.

As natural healers, we work with the magical healing forces of nature including unlimited energy that can be tapped and directed at will. We must always remember, however, that we are only the conduit or the messenger. We are not the energy or the force behind it. Consequently, we should humbly ask the assistance of nature and thank the forces of nature for the gifts we are given to use.

Proper Technique:

In energy healing, it is important to be cautious about applying undue amounts of stress on a healing subject. A little bit of healing energy goes a long way, though the effects may not be obvious. Excessive amounts of energy—say more than 15 minutes of healing at a time, may stress a subject. It is a little like the blazing power of sunlight on the beach. A little feels great and rejuvenates you, but more than that will probably burn you to a crisp. It is better to get a little energy every so often. Healing sessions can be conducted a couple times every day, for instance, as long as no one session is too long or intensive.

Another potential problem with empathic healing technique involves inadequate preparation. It is extremely important that you prepare yourself for energy healing of any kind by grounding and centering yourself first. Then you need to focus your intent, and drive it with the full power of your will.

It will help you immensely to approach natural healing with creative visualization, picturing in your mind's eye exactly what you want to do from beginning to end. This creates thought forms which are energized and powerful when driven by your will and centered with focused intent. Creative visualization acts as a location beacon to help you find your target. If you do not approach energy healing with focused intent in a state of heightened awareness, you will probably not transfer energy effectively. You will go through the motions without achieving results.

It is important to establish that you are making contact with your ailing subject, as you attempt to send healing energy. You can do this in two ways. First, look for a warm or tingling sensation in your hands, if you are using healing hands. Or you might sense a cold spot or emptiness with your hands, as they trace over the outline of the subject's ailing body. In this way, you are using your own body to measure feedback from the ailing subject. Secondly, you can observe your ailing subject for signs that the healing energy you are sending is received and felt. This is easier with people, perhaps, than with pets or plants. People will often comment that they feel a subtle but growing warmness or tingling of some sort when they receive energy from healing hands. Of course, pets might show you with their body language that they are feeling something that is appreciated. Plants might seem to move or tremble with enthusiasm if you watch closely in administering healing touch. It is also possible to receive feedback from your ailing subjects telepathically, as you learn to listen to thought forms in a state of heightened awareness. In the case of healing yourself, you will feel the energy as a warm and tingling sensation in the area of the body where you are directing the energy.

Feedback is more difficult with other forms of healing energy that are not as tactile and direct as healing hands. Nonetheless, you must attempt to establish feedback results through thought forms or a third-party observer, if necessary, to determine that your attempts to direct healing energy to an ailing subject are effective. If not effective, then you need to review the preliminary procedures to establishing a good connection with your subject. It is not necessary that your subject fully believe in the empathic healing process, only that you establish the energy connection.

You must learn to listen with new ears and see with new eyes. That is where heightened awareness comes into play with your new skills of perception. Part of your new set of perceptive skills in heightened awareness is intuition. You must learn to trust this perception. You are working partly outside the ordinary physical reality now in the shadows of the spirit world. The skills of your subtle energy body come into play. You can be keenly observant of the realities that surround the subtle energy bodies, once you learn to meditate properly.

The Proper Use of Healing Energy

Nothing in this book is intended to give you the impression that healing energy or empathic healing is more than a supplement to professional medical care. Every living thing has a right to the best professional medical care it can obtain. Veterinarians train many years to take excellent care of your pet's health. Botanists and professional gardeners are the people to call when your favorite tree is dying or your plants are wilting. On the other hand, empathic healing is a perfectly natural and nurturing response that you can offer your ailing loved ones as a supplement to professional care. Natural healing is the oldest, most time-tested approach to health care and continues to work wonders around the world.

I was hiking with my son once in the national forest at Mount Hood, Oregon, and sprained my ankle coming down the mountain at dusk. We stopped for a minute, so I could remove my shoe. My foot was already swollen so badly from the sprain that I could not put my shoe back on. So I meditated for a minute and then placed my right hand near my swollen ankle. I focused my intent to send healing energy to my swollen ankle. I had never used healing hands on one of my ankles before, but could visualize the healing taking place. In just a few minutes, I felt my ankle beginning to tingle. The fact that it could feel anything besides the throbbing pain seemed to me to be a blessing. To my son's surprise, the ankle swelling decreased in just a couple of minutes to where my hiking shoe fit easily over it and I was able to move quickly down the mountain in the fading light.

Another note about healing energy involves working on difficult cases. It might prove exhausting and frustrating for one person to try to work alone in some situations. I can recall trying to help one friend who was terminally ill with cancer. It was too much to handle. She would drain me quickly and leave me feeling empty—not a good feeling for an empathic healer. So I began working with another friend, who also was trained to use his hands in energy healing. We would work together on the patient at the same time, usually working opposing sides of the body. I might work on the right side, while he worked on the left, all the way down the body. Or he would work the back side, while I worked the front side. This proved very effective.

So when a new friend and I found a badly injured cat in the road outside the Theosophy national headquarters one night, I was so happy that my new friend also was trained somewhat in healing hands and could help me reduce the cat's intense pain at least.

That cat died of complications due to internal injuries and massive trauma, in addition to many broken bones. Sometimes the injuries are just too advanced or severe for the body to rejuvenate, no matter how much energy you use to stimulate their eternal life force. This provides a painful but necessary lesson in the limited application of healing energy for the empathic healer. You cannot be a hero all of the time. In fact, your sharing of energy as an empathic healer makes you only a caring friend who assists another in their natural rejuvenation.

In truth, the natural healer is no hero at all. Sometimes all we can give a loved one is a small gift, like the temporary cessation of pain. For the terminally ill, this might be the greatest gift we can offer—making their final days less painful. That is why energy work, such as healing hands, is appropriate in hospice and nursing home situations.

We must begin to think of the energy we process and transform every day as an abundant gift. In sharing it with others in a natural way, we learn to repay this great gift of spirit.

Bibliography

Andrews, Ted. *Animal-Speak.* St. Paul, Minn.: Llewellyn Publications, 1993.

Barnes, John F. *Myofascial Release I.* Paoli, Penn.: Myofascial Release Treatment Centers and Seminars, 1989.

Brennan, Barbara Ann. *Hands of Light: A Guide to Healing Through the Human Energy Field.* New York, NY: Bantam Doubleday Dell, 1988.

Burns, Echo Bodine. *Hands that Heal.* San Diego, Calif.: ACS Publications, 1985.

Campbell, Don. *The Roar of Silence: Healing Powers of Breath, Tone & Chant.* Wheaton, Ill.: Theosophical Publishing House, 1989.

Carter, Mary Ellen and William A. McCarey. *Edgar Cayce on Healing.* New York, NY: Warner Books, 1972.

Castaneda, Carlos. *Magical Passes: The Practical Wisdom of the Shamans of Ancient Mexico.* New York, NY: HarperCollins Publishers, 1998.

Choa Kok Sui. *The Ancient Science & Art of Pranic Healing.* Quezon City, Metro City, Philippines: Institute for Inner Studies, Inc., 1987.

Choa Kok Sui. *Pranic Psychotherapy.* York Beach, Maine: Samuel Weiser, Inc., 1993.

Conway, D. J. *Animal Magick.* St. Paul, Minn.: Llewellyn Publications, 1995.

Dorosz, Edmund R. *Let's Cook for our Cat.* Fort Macleod, Alberta: Our Pet's Inc., 1995.

Fate Magazine. *Psychic Pets & Spirit Animals.* St. Paul, Minn.: Llewellyn Publications, 1996.

Findhorn Community. *The Findhorn Garden.* New York, NY: Harper & Row, Publishers, Inc., 1975.

Gittner, Louis. *Listen Listen Listen.* Eastound, Wash.: Touch the Heart Press, 1981.

Godwin, Joscelyn. *Harmonies of Heaven and Earth: The Spiritual Dimensions of Music.* Rochester, Vermont: Inner Traditions International, Ltd., 1987.

Heline, Corine. *The Esoteric Music of Richard Wagner.* La Canada, Calif.: New Age Bible & Philosophical Center, 1986.

Hodson, Geoffrey. *Clairvoyant Investigations.* Wheaton, Ill: The Theosophical Publishing House, 1984.

Juhan, Deane. *Job's Body: A Handbook for Bodywork.* Barrytown, NY: Station Hill Press, 1987.

Karagulla, Shafica, and Dora Van Gelder Kunz. *The Chakras & the Human Energy Fields.* Wheaton, Ill.: Theosophical Publishing House, 1998.

Kowalski, Gary. *The Souls of Animals.* Walpole, NH: Stillpoint Publishing, 1991.

Krieger, Dolores. *Living the Therapeutic Touch.* New York, NY: Dodd, Mead & Company, Inc., 1987.

Krieger, Dolores. *The Therapeutic Touch: How to Use Your Hands to Help or to Heal.* New York, NY: Prentice Hall Press, 1986.

Kunz, Dora. *Spiritual Aspects of the Healing Arts.* Wheaton, Ill.: Theosophical Publishing House, 1985.

Lansdowne, Zachary F. Ray *Methods of Healing.* York Beach, Maine: Samuel Weiser, 1993

Lawson, Tony. *The Cat-Lovers' Cookbook.* Avenel, NJ: Wings Books, 1986.

Lingerman, Hal. *The Healing Energies of Music.* Wheaton, Ill.: Theosophical Publishing House, 1995.

McCoy, Edaine. *Entering the Summerland.* St. Paul, Minn.: Llewellyn Publications, 1996.

Miller, Melissa. *The Superior Cat.* New York, NY: Hyperion, 1993.

Morris, Desmond. *Catwatching*. New York, NY: Crown Trade Paperbacks, 1986.

Pitcairn, Richard H. and Susan Hubble Pitcairn. *Dr. Pitcairn's Complete Guide to Natural Health for Dogs & Cats*. Emmaus, Penn.: Rodale Press, Inc., 1995.

Puharich, Andrija. Uri: *The Original and Authorized Biography of Uri Geller – The Man Who Baffled Scientists*. London: W.H. Allen, 1974.

Ray, Barbara. *The Reiki Factor*. St. Petersburg, Florida: Radiance Associates, 1986.

Smith, Penelope. *Animal Talk: Interspecies Telepathic Communication*. Point Reyes Stations, Calif.: Pegasus Publications, 1989.

Smith, Penelope. *Animals...Our Return to Wholeness*. Point Reyes Station, Calif.: Pegasus Publications, 1993.

Steiner, Lee B. *Psychic Self-Healing for Psychological Problems*. Englewood Cliffs, NJ: Prentice-Hall, Inc., 1977.

Stone, Robert B. *The Secret Life of your Cells*. Atglen, Penn.: Whitford Press, 1989.

Tellington-Jones, Linda and Sybil Taylor. *The Tellington T Touch: A Revolutionary Natural Method to Train and Care for Your Favorite Animal*. New York, NY: Penguin Putnam, 1995.

Tompkins, Peter and Christopher Bird. *The Secret Life of Plants*. New York, NY: Harper & Row, Publishers, Inc., 1989.

Tompkins, Peter and Christopher Bird. *Secrets of the Soil: New Solutions for Restoring our Planet*. Anchorage, Alaska: Earthpulse Press, 1998.

Webster, Richard. *Is Your Pet Psychic? Developing Psychic Communication with Your Pet*. St. Paul, Minn.: Llewellyn Publications, 2002.

Special Thanks From the Author

All personal, after-tax profits from the sale of this book will be donated by the author to pet and wildlife charities for badly needed animal care, shelter, and habitat. Thank you for helping to make this possible with your purchase of this book.

Request for responses:

If you have a personal story to tell about your own healing experience with a pet or houseplant and would like to share it, please write to the author for possible inclusion in a sequel edition to this book. Write to:

Von Braschler
c/o Galde Press, Inc.
P.O. Box 460
Lakeville, MN 55044

To order additional copies of this book, please send full amount plus $4.00 for postage and handling for the first book and 50¢ for each additional book.

Send orders to:

Galde Press, Inc.
PO Box 460
Lakeville, Minnesota 55044-0460

Credit card orders call 1–800–777–3454
Phone (952) 891–5991 • Fax (952) 891–6091
Visit our website at http://www.galdepress.com

Write for our free catalog.